# DRIVING WITH CONFIDENCE

## A PRACTICAL GUIDE TO DRIVING WITH LOW VISION

### ELI PELI
*Harvard Medical School, USA*

### DORON PELI

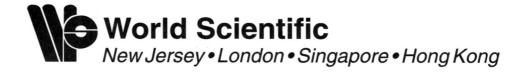
**World Scientific**
*New Jersey • London • Singapore • Hong Kong*

*Published by*
World Scientific Publishing Co. Pte. Ltd.
5 Toh Tuck Link, Singapore 596224
*USA office:* Suite 202, 1060 Main Street, River Edge, NJ 07661
*UK office:* 57 Shelton Street, Covent Garden, London WC2H 9HE

**British Library Cataloguing-in-Publication Data**
A catalogue record for this book is available from the British Library.

This book is NOT a legal document, and
the information contained herein is for
educational purposes only

First published 2002
Reprinted 2003

**DRIVING WITH CONFIDENCE**
**A Practical Guide to Driving with Low Vision**
Copyright © 2002 by World Scientific Publishing Co. Pte. Ltd.

ISBN  981-02-4704-4
ISBN  981-02-4705-2 (pbk)

Printed in Singapore.

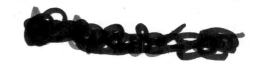

# DRIVING WITH
# CONFIDENCE

## A PRACTICAL GUIDE TO
## DRIVING WITH LOW VISION

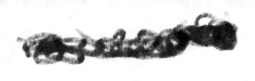

# To Our Parents

# PREFACE

"Driving with Confidence" is not just a catchy title for a book; it is a statement of empowerment. The message is simple: In many cases, persons with low vision conditions can and do receive, retain and exercise their driving privileges, safely, and on a daily basis. Though simple, this message is far from being broadly understood or accepted — in fact, it is quite controversial. This book sheds factual light on the controversy.

America is aging, bringing more and more people into the age group where they have to cope with age-related eye conditions that may interfere with their ability to drive. At the same time, it is these very same new golden-agers who rely and depend on the mobility and freedom provided by driving. "If I was denied driving, I would be furious," says M. S., a low vision driver from New Hampshire. "We live in the country, and if I couldn't drive, I'd be trapped at home."

Many persons with low vision conditions, and even more importantly, many driver licensing authorities, are coming to the realization that driving with low vision is a viable option that should be examined and whenever possible and **safe**, encouraged as another way to enhance and preserve our lifestyle and to exercise our independence. In many states, low vision is no longer a condition that should or could lead to automatic disqualification from driving a car.

Empirical test results could not be clearer: "Students who completed training perform at a level comparable to that of their normally sighted counterparts in terms of basic visual skills in vehicle handling and ability to react to traffic hazards" (Huss, 1996).

Yet, in as many as 20 states, low vision is still a cause for almost certain denial of driving privileges.

This book, co-authored by one of the country's leading low vision rehabilitation experts, contains facts, information, advice and reference materials that will enable those facing a deterioration in their vision to start answering the daunting question: "Is it practical and safe for me to continue driving?" "Driving with Confidence" is also aimed at informing those of us who come in contact with persons with low vision — family members, friends, eye-care professionals, and licensing agency administrators.

A primary mission of this book is to explain that a diagnosis of visual impairment should by no means lead to an automatic decision to give up driving. The proper way to determine fitness to drive is a combination of the assessment of vision disability and the compensatory adaptations as they affect the driving performance of the driver.

"Driving with Confidence" will help you understand your condition, and give you the tools necessary to evaluate your chances of driving safely with impaired vision. We have gathered here a simplified yet comprehensive description of the typical problems faced by drivers with deteriorating vision. We have evaluated the aspects of visual performance needed to ensure safe driving and the visual problems associated with the more common eye diseases.

If you decide to pursue a low vision driver's license "Driving with Confidence" provides structured, practical advice on how to go about resuming or maintaining driving privileges. The book reviews relevant state and federal vision-related licensing regulations, and points the reader to available resources and support services.

At the same time, it is crucial to emphasize that in the first place, it is you, the individual, who must decide whether your days at the wheel are over. This book will help in making this decision an informed one, based on knowledge rather than fear or speculation. If the decision is to quit driving, this book will provide you with specific information on how to organize and finance your transportation needs without a car.

Much of the information on licensing requirements and low vision counseling which you will find in this book is not easily available in one place and in a coherent format and language. We have painstakingly gathered information on vision requirements set by each state's Motor Vehicle Bureau to provide cogent summaries that will be helpful not only to patients, but to ophthalmologists, optometrists, driving instructors, DMV administrators and other specialized professionals who care for and provide services associated with driving and low vision.

And finally, we wish to stress, as we shall do throughout the book, that safety — the public's and the driver's — should always be the overriding consideration in every decision and action relating to driving, and that all low-vision driving-related decisions should be taken only in accordance with local rules and regulations, and only after consultation with and approval by the proper authorities.

# CONTENTS

Contents

# Contents

# CHAPTER 1
# THE FREEDOM TO DRIVE

## DRIVING — A RIGHT OR A PRIVILEGE?

Mobility — the ability to get from point A to point B — is one of the cornerstones of every modern society. And indeed, the freedom to exercise our mobility is a right. In everyday life, for many of us, freedom of mobility translates to our practical dependence on some mode of transportation to get us where we need to go, be it work, shopping, visiting friends or family, taking part in various activities within our community or exploring new places. And with the car as our primary means of transportation, for many driving is not only the means to exercise freedom of mobility, but an integral part of our quality of life.

We take driving so much for granted that we do not realize it is not a right — it is a privilege.

The difference between a right and a privilege is simple: Rights are yours regardless of the will, wishes, opinions or regulations of a government's administrator; privileges are the administrator's to bestow and withhold.

At any given time, your driving privileges can be revoked or revised, and you can be taken off the road, at the discretion of your Department of Motor Vehicle (DMV) administrator based on the rules and regulations enacted by each state's legislator, and the interpretation of these rules by the administrator and its advisory (medical/vision) board.

## DEALING WITH THE THREAT OF LOSING YOUR DRIVING PRIVILEGES

Eye injury or eye disease that affects your vision can jeopardize your freedom to drive, if the administrator decides that the impairment is serious enough to affect your ability to drive safely and legally.

Older people may expect to lose some vision as the years go by. For some the loss is gradual and for others, it may be more abrupt and pronounced. At some point, as a result of such vision loss, you may be faced with a threat to your freedom to drive, previously taken for granted.

Depending on your particular situation such a prospect can be not only frightening but can also threaten your livelihood and your way of life.

Faced with such a threat, some people bow to the inevitable, and though grudgingly, accept and accommodate the loss of the license. Others, on the other hand, insist on challenging administrative decisions, and on examining in detail the legal and medical basis for such decisions.

As a rule, we recommend never to accept the initial determination of the person at the DMV counter as the last and final word on the subject. If you feel that you can drive safely, you should demand and receive full evaluation from your driver's licensing authority.

As we shall see in this book, no two states have an identical set of regulations handling visual requirements for an unrestricted driver's license. The variations are even more pronounced in the way the various states deal with low vision drivers. Vagueness, ambiguity and substantial variations exist between the way that each state deals with drivers and potential drivers with vision impairments. These variations reflect a variety of opinions as well as a measure of confusion as to the question of what should be measured and how, when trying to determine a person's fitness to exercise driving privileges.

But before you go out to argue with the decision makers in your state's Department of Motor Vehicles (DMV), you would want to know everything about your rights and about your limitations: you would most probably want to learn more about your condition, about the rules and regulations governing driving in your state, and about the organizations and professionals that may help you evaluate your condition and decide what to do next.

Alongside your wish to maintain your driving privileges whenever and wherever it is safe and legal to do so, it is also your obligation to consider the eventuality that your vision loss might be of such magnitude or nature so as to prevent you from driving safely. In such a case it would be for your own benefit and everyone else's safety that you quit before a tragedy occurs. Helping you recognize this situation is no less important than helping you stay on the road.

Car accidents take an enormous toll on life, limb and property. In 1996 alone there were about 10 million vehicular collisions in the USA; 41,907 people had died in these crashes, and more than 3.5 millions were injured (Transportation, 1996). Looking at these numbers, it is easy to understand why every decision regarding driving should be taken with the utmost seriousness.

## LOW VISION AND ITS CONSEQUENCES

Low Vision is defined as *vision loss that cannot be corrected by regular spectacles or contact lenses, and is serious enough to be considered disabling.*

The World Health Organization (WHO) classifies the consequences of vision loss in the following way:

*Disorder*
   Deviation from normality in the structure of the eye
      E.g. cataract

*Impairment*
   Limitation in the overall function of the eye
      E.g. reduced visual acuity

*Disability*
   Limitation in the ability to perform a task
      E.g. driving

*Handicap*
  Limitation in the social functioning of a person
    E.g. unable to get to work without driving

A person is considered to have low vision if his vision impairment causes disability.

Vision requirements for driving are typically defined at the impairment level. These requirements are legal terms based on medical measurements. The origin of these requirements is historical and quite arbitrary. Therefore, they vary widely from state to state. Amazingly, none of these requirements were ever shown to be a good predictor of driving performance.

There is a growing recognition among professionals that fitness to drive should be defined at the disability level of the classification. It should be realized that driving permits compensatory approaches on strategic and tactical levels to reduce the disabling effects of the impairment.


## GETTING SOME STRAIGHT ANSWERS FROM YOURSELF AND FROM THE PROFESSIONALS

Trying to decide whether to try and gain or retain driving privileges with vision impairment gives rise to several complex questions about your condition and about what constitutes safe driving. The answers are not always as readily apparent as they may seem at first, and yet the answers you give and receive to these questions may seriously affect your established pattern of life.

Here are some of the questions that you may want to consider, alone, and with the help of professionals, if you are experiencing a deterioration of your vision and are considering its effect on your driving:

■ **Can I continue to drive safely, if I am extra careful?**
  – No, you should immediately consult an eye-care professional.

■ **Must I report my condition to the DMV?**
  – Yes, in many states the law requires that any change in your health be reported.

■ **Whom should I talk to about this?**
  – Your family, your eye-care professional and possibly others. For a detailed list, see Chapter 4.

■ **My license is about to expire. Am I going to be able to pass the vision test?**
  – In many states you can take the test at your eye-care specialist's clinic. If in doubt, take a preliminary test and evaluate your condition together with your specialist.

■ **If my license is suspended or revoked, how should I respond, and how will it affect my life?**
  – The answer to this question is the core of this book.

Obviously, just ignoring the situation would be foolhardy. On the other hand, it could be premature to simply decide to quit driving. Many people in the United States, with reduced vision severe enough to ostensibly fail them in a driving license vision test, DO continue to drive SAFELY AND LEGALLY with the help of appropriate vision aids, counseling and training.

Balancing the individual rights of many thousands of low-vision drivers to enjoy the mobility afforded by a car, against the genuine requirements for public (and personal) safety is neither simple, nor easy. The more information you will collect on these matters, the more educated your decision-making process is likely to be.

"I never questioned my ability to drive (with my condition), but I also did not try to drive beyond my ability," said M. B., a 51 year old bioptic telescope driver with 35 years of low vision driving experience.

No driver, no matter how skilled or hawk-eyed, is guaranteed an accident-free driving record. Accumulated accident statistics have demonstrated that many vision-impaired persons can drive just as safely or even safer than other driver groups. The licensing regulations in many states now reflect this reality.

It is important to recognize that failure to pass the customary vision test used for screening drivers at the time of licensing (usually, the ability to read certain lines of letters on a chart) is not sufficient by itself to demonstrate that an individual cannot drive a car safely. Many states recognize this, and will grant a license based on additional input, although sometimes with restrictions. In states such as Alabama, Arizona, California and New York — to name just a few, applicants for a driver's license who do not pass their first vision screening are allowed to submit the results of a vision screening test conducted by an eye care professional.

Nor, in fact, does the ability to pass a conventional driver's license vision test serve as a guarantee that an individual's vision meets all the needs for driving — as will be discussed later in this book. Passing the DMV's screening test after your eye doctor told you that you lost peripheral vision (peripheral field), should not be considered an assurance of your qualification to drive safely. The proper test may not have been administered, or it may have missed the loss that your doctor diagnosed. It is important to consider your doctor's recommendation and follow-up on it even if you passed the screening test. Otherwise, you may be risking yourself and others.

Many studies have shown that there is very little correlation between safe driving experience and the screening test, when considered by itself (Charman, 1997).

The first good news is that spectacles or contact lenses can frequently improve vision. Careful evaluation of the required spectacle correction may be all that is needed by many. A change in the required spectacle correction is very common in elderly people even if the prescription was stable for many years. Vision loss can also result from eye diseases which, although they can occur at any age, are much more common among older persons. Indeed, one can expect some loss of vision with advancing age, even if there is no evidence of disease requiring medical attention.

⇨ **Remember:** Millions of people in the US have moderately-reduced vision, which may lead to or contribute to failing the driving screening vision tests.

Yet, with today's Low Vision aids, training and legislation, a lot can be done to assist many of these people in regaining the acuity, field of vision and the skills required to legally and safely exercise their driving privileges.

In Chapter 2, we will help you establish a firm understanding of the complex issues involved in low vision and driving. We shall look at some of the more prevalent myths regarding low vision and driving. We will compare the myths to the actual findings of scientific studies. We will also look at the relations between vision and age, and examine the aspects of vision that effect driving.

# CHAPTER 2
# VISION AND DRIVING —
# FACTS AND FICTION

## SIFTING FACTS FROM MYTHS

Misconceptions and myths often cloud the facts and realities of driving with low vision. In this chapter, we shall describe some of the prevailing and sometimes inaccurate popular beliefs associated with low vision and driving. We shall set the record straight and provide you with the sources and the data you need to feel confident when considering your condition and when discussing driving and low vision with friends, colleagues and/or professionals.

## What happens to vision as you age?

Aging brings with it a slow but inevitable loss of some physical capabilities, often including a decline in the quality of vision.

Some vision changes that come with age are considered normal. Most people first notice aging-related visual loss around the age of forty, when reading fine print may become more difficult than before. This normal loss of focusing ability usually can be overcome with bifocals or simple reading glasses. Later on, the pupils of the eyes become smaller. This reduces the amount of light entering the eye, and thus an older person needs more light to see than a younger one. This change in the pupils may also affect the ability to detect objects at night. Note, however, that smaller pupils only reduce the brightness of what is seen, they do not restrict the field-of-view, just as changing the aperture of a camera does not change the field of the picture, only its brightness. Changes such as the diminution of pupil size have a minimal effect on vision in most circumstances and are considered normal aging effects. Small pupils may, however affect driving at night or at dusk.

Oddly enough, this condition has some positive side effects; smaller pupils improve the depth-of-focus and thus the sharpness of vision, when the light is bright. Therefore, it is assumed that the smaller pupils represent a positive adaptation to the degradation of the optical quality of the eyes with the years. But the improvement comes at the price of a small reduction in night vision.

There are other, less subtle, vision changes that show up with age, or are very closely correlated with age — for example, cataracts. Cataracts, the loss of clarity of the eye's lens, almost invariably become more severe with age. Although some young people and even babies may have cataracts, this is rare. Most people develop some cataracts in the course of normal aging. Cataracts may be more consequential for driving, even though you may not immediately recognize a significant problem with your vision or with your eye health. Cataracts may cause an increase in glare from oncoming cars' headlights when driving at night.

Many of the eye diseases that affect driving, such as Glaucoma, Macular Degeneration, and Diabetic eye disease also occur more frequently and with greater severity with increasing age.

In any event, with every change in vision or in the health of the eyes, an eye examination and an evaluation by an eye doctor are essential as a primary basis for assessing the situation.

## Driving-affecting Visual/Perceptual Functions

Many aspects of vision can affect your driving, not just those revealed by the ability to read letters on the eye chart. It is important that you be aware of them, whether or not they are tested as part of your visual screening procedure, and whether or not deficiencies are detected.

Below, we list several aspects of visual performance that are of importance to driving:

■ **Visual Acuity** — This is a measure of the size of the smallest (high contrast) letter/object that you can see and recognize.

■ **Visual Field** — This is a measure of your peripheral vision. It is a measure of how far you can see objects that are off to the side of your direct line of view.

■ **Color Vision** — This is a measure of how well you can distinguish between colors, particularly red and green.

12

- **Contrast Sensitivity** — This is a measure of the ability to detect low contrast stripes of different sizes. Sometimes, it is measured by the ability to read large letters of low contrast.

- **Glare** — This is a measure of how bright light, both during daylight and at night, affects your ability to see and to drive safely.

Because driving is such a complex skill, it is affected not only by the very basic sensory functions described above but also by higher visual information-processing skills such as attention and processing speed. In particular, a reduction in the useful field of view was found to be associated with increased car crash frequency.

- **Useful Field of View** — This is a measure of the visual field area over which one can process visual information that is presented rapidly and simultaneously in more than one place.

## Visually impaired people can drive — safely

Before we start looking at the specific elements of driving and vision we would like to stress one very important point: Many visually impaired people can drive — safely.

"I drove my whole life, using my common sense as my best guide," said S. B., a bioptic telescope driver from Rhode Island.

One of the most popular, and unfortunately most readily accepted and propagated misconceptions about visually-impaired persons, is that they are by far the most dangerous drivers on the road — a real menace to self and public, and one that should be dealt with quickly and sternly. The logic behind this misconception is seemingly iron-clad: Vision is crucial for driving; if you cannot see well, you cannot drive well. Not seeing well is usually associated with reduced visual acuity.

### The facts

The best way to counter the above misconception is with facts. Several studies, which directly examined the relationship between low vision and driving, have shown that although vision is important to driving, poor or imperfect vision is not the major cause of most accidents.

A study by a vision scientist showed that drivers with poor visual acuity did not have worse driving records than those with normal vision. The study, which included a large number of drivers in California, concluded that: "The relationship between the driving record and corrected vision were quite small and in the opposite direction from the expected one, i.e., good vision is associated with a poorer driving record" (Burg, 1967). This indicates that factors other than vision, such as poor judgment, overconfidence and greater risk-taking tendencies may be more conducive to unsafe driving.

A review of the literature relating to driving with visual impairments concluded that: "...Visually impaired individuals are frequently denied licensure due to their inability to satisfy the high visual acuity standards established by regulatory agencies nationwide. This is in spite of the fact that studies comparing the driving records of various groups of handicapped drivers consistently report a favorable ranking of visually impaired drivers" (Appel *et al.*, 1990).

Another paper by vision scientists reported little correlation between vision and driving violations.

"...studies of visual functions and driving performance found little or no relationship between driving accidents and conviction records and different visual parameters" (Keltner and Johnson, 1987). A significant correlation was found in that study only in cases where visual field was severely reduced in both eyes (more than half the visual field was lost).

The most dangerous drivers (higher accident rates) are young men, who typically have excellent vision, but exhibit poor judgment on the road.

Similar failure to find significant correlation between vision and driving performance was the main finding in most studies on the subject presented in the most recent international scientific conference on Vision in Vehicles held in Boston MA in August 1999.

## A focus on visual acuity

Having dealt with the myth of the dangerous visually impaired driver, we can examine in detail several visual aspects of driving, such as visual acuity, peripheral vision, color vision, and others.

## *What is "20/20"?*

We are all aware of the importance of sharpness of vision in driving a car. Vision should be sharp enough to discern detail ahead of us on the road. It is especially important in enabling us to read signs at a distance, particularly warning signs. For example, while driving on a highway, it is important to be able to clearly read the exit signs in time to plan and execute a safe departure from the main road to the secondary, slower, exit road.

The technical term for this aspect of vision is **Visual Acuity**.

Visual acuity is measured by the ability to read letters on the eye chart in the doctor's office. Normal visual acuity is designated by the quotient **20/20**, which is read "twenty-twenty" A person with 20/40 (twenty-forty) acuity can only read letters that are twice as large as those read by a person with a 20/20 acuity. In most states, a visual acuity of 20/40 is required to pass the eye chart test used to screen drivers applying for a license.

The big letter E at the top of a traditional eye chart corresponds to a visual acuity of 20/200.

Individuals who, even with their best regular spectacles, can only read the top E, are considered under federal and most states laws as legally blind, and are often entitled to special assistance and services, including tax advantages. A person who is legally blind due to visual acuity problems may qualify to drive legally in some states, given proper visual aids, training and evaluation, although often with some restrictions, such as daytime driving only.

## 20/40 is NOT the key number

Many individuals, both professionals and laypersons, believe that a visual acuity measure of better than 20/40 is the most significant factor influencing driving safety.

While visual acuity is important to driving, there is growing recognition that the visual acuity requirements set by each state's licensing body are not based strictly on knowledge and understanding, but are to some extent a result of tradition and unsubstantiated beliefs.

A quick glance through each state's visual acuity licensing requirements (Appendix E) reveals an amazing fact: while all states accept visual acuity of 20/40 as sufficient for unrestricted license, almost no two states have the same visual acuity requirements for people not meeting that standard. What better proof that there is no consensus on the visual acuity actually necessary to drive safely! The lack of consensus is due to an absence of substantial, irrefutable data in this field, which has resulted in a multitude of arbitrarily determined standards. If there was one set of numbers that most of the administrative and scientific communities agreed on, it is likely that many licensing bodies would have adopted it, or at least stuck close to the recommended range in their screening procedures.

## The facts

Review paper after review paper (Appel *et al.*, 1990); (Demers-Turco, 1996); (Charman, 1997) highlights the ambiguity, which plagues visual acuity standards. This is an ambiguity that a regulating body can ill afford, but for which no better solution has yet been suggested.

"Recent reports in the ophthalmic and optometric literature suggest that a 20/20-20/40 level of visual acuity is not as important for safe driving as state laws appear to indicate. Fonda and Weiss maintain that the 20/40 requirement is arbitrary and is not based on actual visual acuity demands while driving. Fonda maintains that a person with 20/200 daytime visual acuity, traveling at 40 mph, can recognize a **STOP** sign in sufficient time to react safely" (Appel *et al.*, 1990). Furthermore a recent review of studies on vision impairment and driving (Owsley and McGwin, 1999) notes that "There is remarkable agreement among studies that visual acuity is only weakly associated with crash involvement and unsafe driving performance".

## Static and dynamic acuity

If more proof is needed that the question of the necessity of visual acuity for safe driving remains largely unresolved today, consider the question of static versus dynamic acuity.

Many people believe that the **static acuity** test, the traditional "Stand in front of the board, cover one eye at a time and read the letters from top to bottom" screening performed by most DMVs — where the patient and the targets are stationary — is the most relevant test for identifying vision problems while driving. However, all the research to date fails to support this belief.

Since most driving involves being in motion, it is reasonable to assume that what really counts when you drive is what you see on the move — **Dynamic Acuity**. Yet not a single state's DMV administers Dynamic Acuity tests to potential drivers. At the same time, the test for Static Acuity, the famous 20/20 test, is the most prevalent visual screening test given today to prospective drivers.

## *The facts*

The paper quoted below implies that if we want to really do something about screening for potential visual acuity problems in driving, we ought to screen for Dynamic Acuity. Yet we do not!

"Research by Burg has shown that accident rates have a 10 times higher correlation with Dynamic Acuity (Dynamic acuity is measured when the patient is stationary and the targets are moving)" (Appel *et al.*, 1990).

Why don't we test for Dynamic Visual Acuity? The reason is that even with this higher correlation, the correlation is still too small for scientists to be able to predict with reasonable confidence an individual's ability to drive safely, based on his/her visual acuity test results — Static or Dynamic. Thus, adding this complex and expensive test will yield no benefit to public safety (Charman, 1997).

## Peripheral vision/visual field

In order to see clearly, we must point our eyes and aim them *directly* at the object of our interest. As we do this, we are able at the same time to take in visual information from a very wide field of view on either side of that object, and perceive both motion and other objects in the periphery of our vision.

This ability to see things off to the side is referred to as **peripheral vision**.

The extent of our peripheral vision is measured by the visual field of each eye, and expressed as a visual angle. For example: When you hold your hand in front of your face, stretched at arm length, the four fingers span about 5 degrees of visual angle. If while looking straight ahead, you are able see both your hands as you raise them from the side of your body to your shoulders height pointing sideways, your visual field is 180 degrees.

It is important to realize that the visual fields of both eyes are highly overlapping. Therefore, a loss of field in one eye has only a minimal impact on the visual field of the person. This is why all states permit people with one blind eye to drive, although many require the remaining eye to satisfy a higher standard on vision tests than that required from people with two functioning eyes. In some countries an adaptation period of a few months is required before driving is resumed after a loss of vision in one eye.

A visual field of 100 degrees or more, along the horizontal dimension, is required for driving in many states. Whether required by law or not, an adequate visual field is clearly important for safe driving. This is the aspect of vision that enables us to detect the presence of an object at the side of the road even though our vision may be directed to the car in front of us. Peripheral vision also allows us to detect moving objects off to the side, a valuable capability in an emergency. For example: It is your peripheral vision, which is most likely to help you notice a child chasing after a ball **BEFORE** the child runs into the street; and it is your peripheral vision that lets you see a car overtaking you when you consider changing a lane.

Peripheral vision is much less sharp than vision straight ahead, but it is extremely important to the overall visual function.

Certain eye diseases, such as Retinitis Pigmentosa (RP) and Glaucoma, can result in a severely restricted visual field, often known as "tunnel vision." Such a condition can greatly affect safe mobility even on foot, let alone during driving.

To appreciate the importance of peripheral vision, try viewing the world through a paper-towel cardboard tube. This simulates extreme loss of visual field (tunnel vision). Hold the tube right in front of one eye, and with the other eye shut look around and consider how difficult it would be to walk even from one room to another room in a safe familiar place like your home.

A person is considered legally blind when his/her visual field is reduced to 20 degrees or less, even if visual acuity is 20/20. An eye doctor using standard instruments can accurately measure the visual field.

Thirty-six of the states require prospective drivers to undergo a peripheral vision screening and a few of them require this type of screening only from those applying for a commercial driver license (bus, taxi, or truck drivers). It is interesting to note that the federal requirement for commercial drivers is for a field of 70 degree horizontally in each eye, considerably less than the requirement imposed by most states for professional or private drivers. The states can and do require in many cases a higher standard than the minimum imposed by the federal regulation.

While it is quite clear that a person who is legally blind due to visual field restriction could not drive safely, it is far less clear what size of the visual field would be consistent with safe driving. A number of studies found no correlation between crash rate and visual field deficits (Decina and Staplin, 1993); (Ball *et al.*, 1993); (Burg, 1967). One study did find a doubling of crashes and traffic violations in people with severely reduced visual field in both eyes (Johnson and Keltner, 1983). Studies conducted in driving simulators or a closed driving course, using simulated visual field defects in people with normal sight, are also less than conclusive with regards to the effect on driving performance and are considered by most as less than relevant.

An extensive review of the literature on the subject, conducted in 1985, concluded that the findings are inconclusive with regards to the impact of field defects on driving safety (North, 1985). The lack of conclusive scientific data and therefore agreement on this subject results in highly variable visual field requirements even between states that have such requirements. While, some states require a field as wide as 140 degrees others are satisfied with as little as 60 degrees or even 35 degrees. Charman (1997) in a review of vision and driving similarly reported that some studies have found some correlation between visual field loss due to RP and others (even by the same authors) fail to find such correlation. A more recent review of the literature on vision impairment and driving (Owsley and McGwin, 1999) determined that "The most prudent conclusion based on the literature may be that, although severe binocular visual field loss elevates crash risk, more subtle visual field impairment by itself is not likely to play a significant role in adverse driving events".

It is clear also that to some extent eye and head movements can compensate for visual field loss. It would be important to determine which driver can apply such compensations effectively in deciding about licensing. This is again a place where the level of disability rather than the impairment, currently being measured, may be more relevant.

Hemianopia, the loss of half the visual field on one side in both eyes, is a distinct type of vision loss that should be considered separately from the peripheral field constriction of RP and Glaucoma. Unfortunately, hemianopia's effect on driving is not distinguished from other types of field loss. For example, the study of Johnson and Keltner (1983), which evaluated 20,000 drivers, is frequently cited as indicating that hemianopia may be dangerous. But according to Dr. Johnson very few people (only two) with hemianopia were included in this study. It is important to realize that not all patients with hemianopia fail to qualify for a driver's license in all jurisdictions. Further, some recovery of visual field is not rare, and with time a person that fails to meet the requirements may exhibit sufficient improvement to qualify again. A Canadian study (Parisi *et al.*, 1991) found that while 34 patients out of 60 with hemianopia failed to meet their province's visual field requirements on initial presentation, 20 of them presented sufficient improvement to pass a follow-up test about two years later.

Most studies on hemianopia and driving were conducted in driving simulators. A Swedish study (Lovsund *et al.*, 1991) evaluated 31 patients with visual field defects (15 of them with hemianopia). The study found that only four of those tested compensated sufficiently for loss of normal performance. The driving task in the study was extremely difficult (driving at 60 mph on a two lane road), and the participants had to respond to very small targets. In fact, it is impressive that four patients with field loss could perform that well in that study. A more recent simulator study compared six patients with hemianopia to a similar number of normally sighted subjects of similar age, and to young drivers. The patients with hemianopia performed worse than the normally sighted ones on a few measures (lane boundary crossing and lane position), but were not different on seven other measures. More importantly, simulator accidents occurred only with two of the normally sighted control subjects. A recent road driving study in Holland resulted in a driver's license being awarded by the local authorities to six out of 30 hemianopia patients.

It is clear that not all people with hemianopia function at the same level, and many probably could not drive safely. However, a fair percentage of these patients may compensate for their visual loss to such an extent that they can drive as safely as any driver. Currently, only a few states provide a road test or evaluation for these patients, and there are no states that officially recognize the use of visual aids for visual field defects.

## Color vision and driving

Color vision refers to the ability of the eye to distinguish between objects of different color.

The common term "color blind" is usually a misnomer, since it implies a complete inability to distinguish colors, an extremely rare condition. Most commonly, color vision deficiency results in some difficulty to distinguish between the colors red and green.

This is, of course, of some importance for drivers. If this inability results in a mismatch in selecting clothing there may be a minimum of risk to health and safety. But the same problem can lead to a real risk for a driver who cannot distinguish between red and green traffic lights.

"The only place where I feel some apprehension (during driving) is when I approach traffic lights," says S. B., a veteran bioptic telescope driver from Rhode Island.

Significant color vision deficiency is usually genetic in origin, and is more common in men. About 10% of all men and 0.5% of women have some kind of color vision deficiency. Many tests are available for eye doctors to evaluate color vision. Very few eye diseases cause color vision deficiencies.

An extensive review of the scientific literature on color vision and driving (Vingrys and Cole, 1988) found that in the vast majority of studies, no association was reported between color vision deficiencies and crash involvement or driving performance. Only nineteen states require prospective drivers to undergo color vision screening. Most of them restrict this requirement to commercial drivers only. In some states, low vision drivers are tested for color vision. Some states require drivers to have normal color vision. Others require only the ability to distinguish red from green.

In most states, a standardization of the traffic lights with the red light on top reduces the importance of color vision in interpreting the color signals. Most drivers consider the top light in a light signal to be the stop signal, and the bottom light to be the go signal. A color-blind person can see which of the lights is on, even if he/she cannot name the color. A new type of traffic lights, using the more efficient and reliable light emitting diodes (LED) is now under consideration. Some of these designs will have only one fixture for all three lights and may prove problematic for visually impaired color deficient drivers.

## Contrast sensitivity

Contrast sensitivity is a measure of the ability to see low contrast objects both large and small. Contrast sensitivity to small objects is highly related to visual acuity. The ability to see much larger objects of very low contrast could be unrelated to visual acuity, yet may be quite relevant to driving tasks. For example, the ability to spot a dark-color car against the dark asphalt of a road, or a white car on a snow-covered road may be assessed by contrast sensitivity measurements. A number of studies reported association between reduced contrast sensitivity and either poor performance in driving test, increased reports of driving difficulties, and, possibly, higher involvement in at-fault car crashes (Wood and Troutbeck, 1992);

(Rubin *et al.* 1994); (Ball *et al.*, 1993). At the moment, no state requires contrast sensitivity testing for driving license qualification.

## The glaring dangers of glare

Glare from the sun or from vehicles' headlights may be the cause of many accidents, and the effects of glare are more severe for elderly drivers. Most drivers experience some difficulty or discomfort from glare when driving towards a low, rising or setting sun in the morning or evening, or at night from oncoming headlights. "I found out that driving during high-glare hours (morning and dusk) and during periods when shadows are long (morning and dusk) is more difficult for me, and I decided to schedule my trips to avoid driving during these periods," say M. S., a bioptic telescope driver from New Hampshire.

As we shall see, with some eye diseases the sensitivity to glare increases considerably. This can be very disabling, and lead to hazardous situations when driving.

It is especially important for drivers with vision disability to acquire skills in selecting and properly using sunglasses or the car's overhead visors, and in avoiding driving in situations where glare may be detrimental to safe driving. Extra attention to windshield cleanliness is also needed.

There are no well-accepted routine tests for measuring sensitivity to glare. The states do not mandate tests to evaluate the effects of glare, either from the sun or from other cars at night.

For additional information regarding Glare and Glare Control, please refer to Appendix C — Glossary.

## Useful Field of View

The Useful Field of View (UFOV) examination tests the ability of an observer to process information presented rapidly in more than one place at the same time and in the presence of distracters. By presenting visual targets under difficult conditions, the area over which a person can direct and divide visual attention may be measured. It was found that these abilities are severely reduced in the elderly, even in the absence of visual impairments (Ball *et al.*, 1990). It was further shown by the same authors that reduction of the UFOV is associated with history of at-fault crash involvement (Owsley *et al.*, 1991); (Owsley and Ball, 1993). A reduction of the UFOV was also found to predict future (three years) crash involvement probabilities (Owsley *et al.*, 1998). These findings suggest that visual attention and the speed of processing may be critical skills for driving and may serve as better screening methods compared with current basic visual function tests. However, at the moment no jurisdiction is applying such tests (UFOV or other) for driving licensing

## How to look at visual screening tests

Visual screening standards are designed to identify drivers and/or potential drivers whose vision is considered by the authorities as sufficient to grant a driver's license without further questions or tests. Screening is also helpful to identify potential drivers whose measured vision parameters fall outside the defined standard, and who may require further testing or evaluation. Visual screening standards are set by each state's legislature and are implemented by the Department of Motor Vehicles (DMV).

In many cases, however, these screening standards are used to unnecessarily deny low vision drivers their driving privileges. This improper use of the screening standard is due to a lack of understanding, by both laypersons and professionals, of the intended purpose of the screening tests. Even persons applying the screening tests frequently do not know that their state laws permit driving (possibly with a restricted license) for people who fail the screening test but who can meet some other standard.

Consider the fact that almost no two states have identical visual licensing standards. Consider also, that (as seen in some of the examples brought up in this book and in many other studies) emerging data disputes what has long been considered the accepted wisdom in many aspects of visual screening and its effectiveness.

Taken all together, we believe that it is proper and necessary to closely examine the validity and utility of these standards and to try to establish proper visual screening as well as procedures to further evaluate drivers who fail these screening tests. In most states, the initial evaluation following such failure will be at your eye-care provider (an ophthalmologist or an optometrist).

⇨ **Remember:** If you were a careful, considerate, defensive and thinking driver, you probably remain so despite losing some of your eyesight.

## Would/Should your eye doctor report your condition to your state-licensing agency?

If your eye care provider finds that you no longer qualify for driving in your state, should he/she report you to the state? This is an important ethical dilemma that bothers many doctors and patients; it is also an important legal question. On the one hand, there is the risk that you may cause harm to yourself and to others. When this serious risk is considered it would seem an ethical imperative for the doctor to inform the state of your disability and help them remove this risk from you and from the rest of society. At the same time, this kind of disclosure has the potential of disrupting the confidential nature of the patient-doctor relationship. Many doctors and patients advocates are concerned that patients with eye diseases might not seek medical care if they feared being turned in by their doctor.

In 1999, a report by the American Medical Association Council on Ethical and Judicial Affairs stated that, if all other interventions fail, reporting an impaired driver to a state licensing agency is both ethical and permissible. For the good of society, the report stated, doctors can, and sometimes should, breach patient confidentiality (Karmel, 2000). Many doctors do not agree with this view and that is why the final recommendation was changed to the word "permissible" from the original recommendation that used the word "mandatory".

The ethics of reporting a patient to the authorities is a difficult question placing many doctors in a difficult dilemma. In addition, one has to consider the legal requirements. While doctors in Canada are required to report patients with physical or mental disability to the licensing agency in all of the provinces, in the USA only a few states place such requirement on the doctor. According to the American Association of Motor Vehicles Administrators report, only California, Nevada, North Dakota, and Texas are known to impose such a requirement (Karmel, 2000).

However, if a doctor chooses to report a patient voluntarily (and most doctors will not do this lightly even with the current ethical permission of the AMA), many states keep the report confidential and protect the reporting doctor's identity. Upon receiving such a report, many states (but not all) will suspend the license. Still, in most cases, additional exams and tests are required before such suspension takes place. Specific information is included in the state-by-state tables of Appendix E. In testing commercial drivers, the federal department of transportation requires that failure to meet the standard will be reported. In this case, however, the driver is referred for additional evaluation, and it is not their own personal doctor who is conducting the evaluation in most cases.

In Chapter 3, we take a close look at the human eye, and provide a detailed description of the more common conditions that may affect your vision and your driving or your chances to receive or maintain a driver's license. Each condition is explained, together with its potential effect on your driving and a discussion of the ways in which you may compensate, if possible, for the condition.

# CHAPTER 3
# THE MEDICAL SIDE OF LOW VISION

## THE EYE

The human eye is a wondrous creation. On the average, the human eye moves about three to five times every second. If we consider the product of each such move as a new image, the human eye feeds the brain about 300 new images every minute.

Obviously, the eyes are **the major** source of information while driving a car. So it is no great surprise that licensing authorities everywhere concentrate their screening efforts around vision. What is surprising is that some crucial elements of vision, such as field of vision and possibly contrast sensitivity, are not always examined thoroughly — if at all.

## How does the eye work?

The human eye is a most efficient and fascinating instrument. The round globe, filled with a gel called the vitreous humor, maintains its spherical shape due to the high fluid pressure inside the eye, just like the pressure of air inside a balloon.

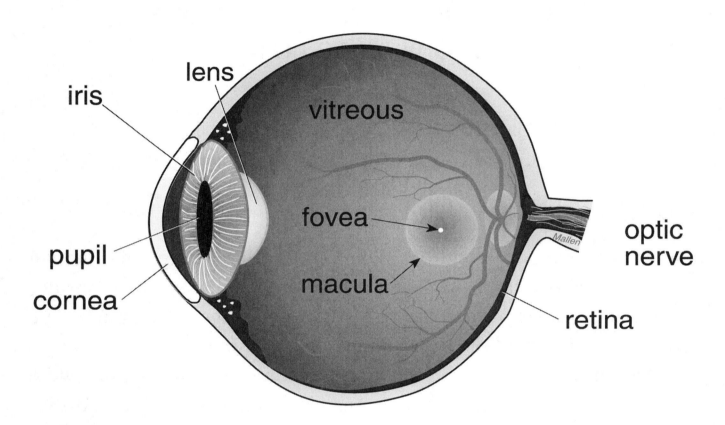

**An illustration of the eye and the parts relevant to the discussion of various diseases below.**

## *The cornea — A window to the world*

The front of the eye is a transparent window called the cornea, which looks like the crystal cover on a watch. In addition to allowing the transmission of light into the eye, the cornea also serves as the main optical element in the eye. It bends the light rays to focus them on the retina at the back of the eye.

## *The crystalline lens — Adjusting the focus*

In addition to the cornea, there is one more lens in the eye's optical system. This one is called the crystalline lens, and it is situated behind the pupil, closer to the front of the eye than to the back. While the crystalline lens has a minor role in focusing the light compared to the cornea, it plays a major role in adjusting the eye's focus between near and far objects. Unfortunately, with the passage of years, the crystalline lens becomes harder and less flexible, and thus it starts to lose its focusing-adjustment ability at around the age of 40. To compensate for this loss, we use reading glasses or bifocals.

The two lenses in the eye, the cornea and crystalline lenses, must stay transparent and clear to facilitate sharp vision. As they are made of live tissue, the maintenance of transparency is a complex and difficult biological task.

When diseases affect the cornea it loses its transparency and becomes cloudy, like ground glass, blurring the vision. Often, such a condition requires a transplant. The crystalline lens gradually loses transparency as it gets harder and loses its flexibility. It too takes on the appearance of ground glass, at which time it is called a cataract. A cataract-affected lens can be removed surgically and replaced with a transparent plastic lens. If the cornea becomes opaque a transplant of a cornea from a human donor may replace it. This is a good reason to consider registering as a tissue donor when you get your driving license.

## *The iris — A colorful peephole*

Between the cornea and the lens we find the iris — the colored portion of the eye. The opening in the center of the iris is called the pupil. The movements of the iris enlarge and shrink the pupil and regulate the amount of light entering the eye. At night, the pupil is wide open to allow the best passage of light into the eye, and in the bright sunlight the pupil contracts to a small diameter, to limit the light entering the eye. The changes in pupil size, to accommodate changes in illumination, take as much as one second to complete. With age, the pupil too loses its flexibility; it becomes smaller than its original adult size, and is less responsive to the change in light intensity. As a result, older people usually have less light available for vision than they actually need to see properly in low-light conditions.

## *The retina — The inner lining*

The retina, the lining of the entire inner rear side of the eye, is an extremely delicate nerve tissue, with the consistency of a wet tissue paper. The images entering the eye through the lenses are projected on the retina and are converted by the retina's light-sensitive detector cells into electrical signals. After some processing in the retinal nerve cells these visual signals are transmitted to the brain, where the perception of images takes place. The retinal signals are transferred to the brain through the optic nerve, starting at the optic-nerve-head — a small opening at the back of each eye globe about 1.5 mm (1/16 of an inch) in diameter.

Inside the eye, the retina covers an area about the size of a US quarter coin. However, only a very small portion of that area is dedicated to processing sharp vision. The central area of the retina, called the Macula, serves that purpose. The Macula is smaller than a dime. In the center of the macula, there is an even smaller area called the Fovea; the Fovea is the size of a pinhead, and it facilitates sharp vision. This area of sharp vision covers a very small portion of the visual world, about the size of one thumbnail held at arm's length. The rest of the retina provides a progressively blurrier vision the farther it is from the Fovea. This blurred peripheral vision is needed to detect objects of interest or obstacles. The movements of the eyes, effectively scanning this tiny area of sharp vision across large areas creates our perception of a clear sharp vision of the world. When the Fovea is damaged, as is the case in a number of diseases, the sharp vision provided by it is lost and vision becomes permanently blurred.

Diseases of the optic nerve, such as glaucoma, and diseases of the retina, such as retinitis pigmentosa, might cause damage first to the peripheral retina outside the Macula. Under these conditions, sharp vision is maintained but the wide field of view provided by the rest of the retina is lost, resulting in **tunnel vision**.

## EYE DISEASES THAT AFFECT YOUR VISION

### Cataract

This is a common condition characterized by a loss of clarity of the crystalline lens within the eye. This causes a general blurring of vision, resulting in a reduction in visual acuity and minimally affects peripheral vision. Seeing through a cataract is similar to looking through a ground glass window; everything appears at a lower contrast and looks less sharp. When bright light impacts a cataract, it causes an effect that we call glare. The glare effect of cataract is more pronounced at night, when light from approaching cars' headlights impacts the lens. Cataracts evolve gradually and are associated with aging. Cataracts will affect almost everyone eventually and with varying results. About half of the people age 75 have early cataracts and a quarter of them have advanced cataracts.

Because a cataract usually progresses slowly, visual disability may advance farther than the patient realizes. One warning sign is the realization when driving that it is becoming gradually more difficult to read street signs, particularly in dim light. People with cataracts complain of driving difficulties, usually avoid difficult situations such as driving at night or in bad weather and sometimes choose to stop driving alltogether. One study found increased risk of car crashes in people with cataracts (Owsley *et al.*, 1999), but two other studies did not find similar increases (McCloskey *et al.*, 1994); (Foley *et al.*, 1995).

When the reduction in vision advances to a point where visual disability becomes a handicap, the affected lens may be removed surgically from the eye and replaced with a plastic lens. In some patients, where the cataract is the only cause of vision loss, this procedure may restore vision (visual acuity) to 20/20. Successful cataract surgery usually removes the driving difficulties caused by the cataracts.

Cataract surgery is a highly perfected procedure, and is usually carried out on an outpatient basis. However, until the cataract is removed, people suffer the disabling effect of the developing cataracts. Unattended, cataract can lead to virtually total blindness. This is common in the third world but rare in the USA.

## Age-Related Macular Degeneration (AMD)

AMD is the most common cause of legal blindness and low vision in the USA. This disease affects the fovea, the very small region (the size of a pinhead) in the center of the retinal area called the macula that provides sharp vision.

With AMD, peripheral vision is unaffected, which means that the patient maintains good mobility, can walk in reasonable safety and possibly even drive. Total blindness is extremely rare with this disease, but the loss of central, sharp, vision means that visual acuity is reduced, often severely.

Patients with macular degeneration frequently have more difficulty and take longer to recover from the glare effect of bright lights. In fact, delayed glare recovery is one of the diagnostic signs of macular degeneration. This may interfere with the night driving of people with macular degeneration, sometimes even before the visual acuity is significantly affected. Some glare control techniques are addressed in Appendix C.

The loss of visual acuity limits the ability of people with AMD to read road signs and traffic signals and to discern details. With advanced AMD there is a blank (light insensitive) region that appears right in the direction of viewing. The patient must learn to make use of the residual functioning peripheral retina to detect and recognize objects. Most people develop this eccentric viewing technique naturally. However, for some it is difficult to master for many months after vision loss in the second eye. Driving should be avoided at least until the eccentric viewing is mastered. However, even with eccentric viewing, the limited resolution capability of the peripheral retina causes blurred vision.

There are two types of AMD, commonly referred to as "dry" and "wet". Most people with AMD have the "dry" type.

The "dry" AMD results in a slow progressive loss of visual acuity. This may develop into the "wet" type, so named because it is characterized by the leakage of fluid (serum or blood) into the retina. The leakage causes damage and rapid visual loss, followed by scarring of the retina that makes the damage permanent. The leakage of fluid and resulting damage can be arrested or slowed by laser treatment in some cases. Currently, there is no treatment for "dry" AMD.

The loss of visual acuity for distant objects may be compensated for by the use of a spectacle-mounted telescope referred to as a 'bioptic telescope'. This small telescope is mounted on the upper region of the spectacle lens, and gives a magnified image. Bioptic telescopes can be focused for use at different distances, and are useful for many activities in addition to driving (i.e., watching TV, movies, or sports as well as hobbies and work). Bioptic telescopes are permitted for driving in many states (see Appendix E).

## Glaucoma

Glaucoma is a disease of the optic nerve, which is frequently (but not always) associated with elevated pressure of the fluids inside the eye.

The damage to the optic nerve results in a loss of the eye's visual field, which begins usually unnoticed, in the outer portions of the peripheral visual field. Glaucoma is an insidious disease, since it progresses so slowly that the patient may be unaware of any vision loss until the condition is advanced.

Early detection is important, since the disease can be controlled — though not cured — in the early stages, usually with the aid of eye drops. Some types of rare glaucomas can be treated and some may be even cured with laser or surgery.

Detection of glaucoma is most commonly achieved using the pressure test, which is a part of routine eye exams, combined with tests of visual fields and observation of the optic nerve through the pupil. The loss of peripheral vision associated with Glaucoma may significantly affect driving safety. A full-blown, mature and uncontrolled Glaucoma may result in total blindness.

## Diabetic Retinopathy

The name of this condition means a degeneration of the retina, caused by diabetes. The visual loss caused by this disease ranges from moderate to very severe. Control of sugar level in the blood and proper diet can postpone the onset of diabetic retinopathy.

Many years of diabetes may lead to damage to the small blood vessels in the retina, which, in turn may result in leakage of serum or blood into the fluid filling the eyeball. The leaking serum causes macular edema (swelling of the retina) that leads to moderate blurring of vision, similar to that caused by cataracts. Diabetes-related macular edema can be treated effectively using lasers. As many as 3000 laser burns are applied to the retinal periphery in a procedure called pan retinal photocoagulation (PRP). While each laser burn is small and its effect on vision in the periphery is minimal, the accumulated effect of a large number of burns results in a significant visual field loss. A number of studies showed that large percentage of patients undergoing this procedure may fail the visual field test required for driving (Mackie *et al.*, 1995); (Pearson *et al.*, 1998). Thus, patients who have been successfully treated with PRP should carefully evaluate their fitness to drive due to the field loss, even if the treatment made it possible for them to pass the visual acuity test at the DMV.

At the later stage of the disease, small, fragile blood vessels may form and these may bleed inside the eye. Internal bleeding usually causes an immediate and severe visual loss. Subsequent scarring, which occurs when the body repairs the effects of the bleeding, may cause further damage to the retina. These new blood vessels can be treated with laser as well. This treatment is successful usually, and typically does not cause any visual deficit that may affect driving.

## Retinitis Pigmentosa (RP)

RP is a group of degenerative diseases that cause deterioration of the retina. It is an inherited condition, and it usually starts affecting vision during the teenage years. The reasons for the onset of this disease are not fully understood. What is known is that the rod-shaped photoreceptor cells in the retina slowly stop functioning in patients with RP. Both peripheral vision and night vision depend on the proper functioning of the rods. As the disease progresses over the years, peripheral vision diminishes, leaving only the very central area functioning. As the field of vision narrows (tunnel vision), it becomes increasingly difficult to detect and avoid obstacles, and this may lead to a need to use a long (white) cane. In most cases the disease progresses further to affect the central vision as well, leading to total vision loss. The affected person loses the ability to see, first in the dark (night blindness), and later, as the disease gradually progresses, it affects peripheral vision, reducing the field of vision. This, in turn, may affect the ability to drive safely, even before the damage is detected. RP may cause total blindness. In some cases, it is also associated with deafness (Usher's Syndrome).

## Optic Atrophy

This is a condition characterized by a degeneration of the optic nerve — the nerve that conducts the visual signals from the eye to the brain. This condition may be caused by Multiple Sclerosis (MS), small strokes (clotting or bleeding) in the nerve itself, or by a general, small blood-vessel disease. The disease results in immediate, sometimes extensive, loss of vision in the center of the eye. Usually one eye is affected first and then the other. Usually the vision loss associated with optic atrophy is too severe to support driving.

## Corneal Dystrophy

This condition is also characterized by opacification (loss of clarity) in the front of the eye — the visible, transparent cornea in front of the pupil. The effects of this condition on vision are similar to those of a cataract. In severe cases, a transplant of a clear cornea from a donor's eye may replace the diseased cornea. This transplant is frequently successful in restoring sight. In severe cases when the transplant is rejected, a plastic implant may restore vision.

A very mild corneal haze may be caused by the laser surgery used to correct shortsightedness. This haze also causes glare problem similar to the glare caused by cataracts and corneal dystrophies, although less severe. It is interesting to note that Canada's Department of Health recommended recently that people undergoing such laser refractive surgery should take night vision tests before a driving license is granted (Hilton, 2001). At the same time, pilots in the US Army are permitted to undergo this procedure.

## Stroke (Hemianopia)

This disease is characterized by a loss of half of the visual field in both eyes, resulting in total vision loss to the right or left of the eye's mid-line. This condition is a result of loss of function on one side of the visual brain, caused by strokes, brain surgery to remove tumors, or head trauma (frequently caused by car accidents). The visual loss on one side of the eye may cause the patient to miss objects on that side, and may result in bumping into obstacles when walking. Obviously, driving with this condition may be dangerous, though the evidence for that is limited as discussed later. Optical devices (prisms and mirrors) may be used to enlarge the visual field, but they are not explicitly approved for driving in any state.

Although many vehicle-licensing authorities do not test visual field during license renewal, no one with hemianopia should drive without being evaluated and approved by professional driving examiners. In particular, some patients with hemianopia suffer from spatial neglect as well. These patients are completely unaware of the space on one side of their body and thus cannot drive safely.

In the next chapter, we provide a structured approach designed to help you make an educated decision on whether you wish to drive with a low vision condition. Assuming you have decided to go ahead and get a driver's license, we will guide you through the steps that we think will facilitate the safe and organized process required to achieve your goal.

# CHAPTER 4
# THINKING ABOUT DRIVING

## MAKING AN INFORMED DECISION

A decision by a person with a low vision condition to retain, renew or try to receive a driver's license is not an easy one, and rightly so. It is crucial that such a decision is arrived at with the maximum amount of knowledge.

Before you start down the road to getting your driver's license, take the time to ask yourself and others some important questions. Try to consult with as many people as possible. Exchange views with your family, vision care and health care professionals, and collect as much information as possible before making up your mind and setting on the path to realizing your wishes.

## A QUICK SELF-TESTING QUESTIONNAIRE

If you are not entirely certain of your suitability to drive a car with your low vision condition, answer the following questionnaire.

While these questions do not cover all the issues relevant to your decision, they contain some guidelines to help you make up your mind.

**Note:** If you are not currently driving, you can take a ride with a friend and find out the answers to most of the questions below from the passenger seat.

1. **Do you have difficulties reading clearly and rapidly all the instruments on a car's dashboard?**
   - In daylight — Yes / No
   - In dim light (dawn, dusk, heavy clouds) — Yes / No
   - At night — Yes / No

2. **Do you have difficulties reading road signs, or if you are currently driving, do you notice and understand the signs in time to react to them with comfort?**
   - In daylight — Yes / No
   - In dim light (dawn, dusk, heavy clouds) — Yes / No
   - At night — Yes / No

3. **Do other cars on the road appear to "pop" into and out of your field of vision unexpectedly?**
   - Yes / No

4. **If you are currently driving — while on the road, do you drive well below the speed limit and slower than most cars around you?**
   - In daylight — Yes / No
   - In dim light (dawn, dusk, heavy clouds) — Yes / No
   - At night — Yes / No

**5. If you are currently driving — do you have difficulties positioning yourself on the road, with respect to other cars, lane markers, curves, sidewalks, parking spaces etc.?**

- In daylight — Yes / No
- In dim light (dawn, dusk, heavy clouds) — Yes / No
- At night — Yes / No

**6. Do you find yourself feeling confused and/or disoriented on the road?**

- In daylight — Yes / No
- In dim light (dawn, dusk, heavy clouds) — Yes / No
- At night — Yes / No

## How to interpret your answers

### *If you currently drive*

If you answered **Yes** to **ANY** of the above questions, you may want to suspend your driving until you consult a specialist. If your answers indicate that you may have a problem under certain conditions (i.e., dim light or night) you may want to suspend your driving under those conditions until you consult a specialist further.

### *If you are not currently driving*

Again, if you answered YES to any of the questions, you should discuss your condition with a low-vision specialist. A thorough examination of your eyes will probably tell you whether you should continue pursuing a driver's license or look into other alternatives (see Chapter 8).

⇨ **Remember:** In most states, you **must** report to your local DMV any change in your health or mental condition, including changes in vision. In a few states your doctor is obliged to report you to the DMV (see Appendix E).

## WHAT DO YOU NEED TO KNOW?

There are several things you would want to know, and several things you would probably want to do, before you decide to dedicate the time and resources necessary to get you on the road or keep you there.

The main things you want to know are:

- Know everything you can about your condition.
- Know the laws and regulations governing low vision driving in your state, and in other states.
- Know the latest medical/technical developments associated with low vision and driving.
- Know who plays a role in your quest for a driver's license.

### Know your medical condition

The best way to get a clear picture of your condition is to collect all pertinent data from your eye specialist, ophthalmologist or optometrist, neurologist, or from any other relevant professional who has been involved in giving you eye care of any sort.

Before embarking on the road to acquiring or retaining your driving license, you should also undergo a thorough physical checkup.

The purpose of the physical checkup is to make sure that no other condition will interfere with or exacerbate your condition, or prevent you from getting your driver's license.

Contact your health service providers, tell them about your plans, share with them your thoughts, and feelings, and encourage them to give you as informative and as detailed feedback as possible.

This is also a good opportunity for you to make sure again that you are aware of and are willing to work hard to acquire, sharpen and continuously improve those physical and mental skills which you will need to drive safely.

There may also be some financial outlay to cover cost of visual aids and training. Neither of these is usually covered by health insurance.

After you have gathered all the pertinent information, you need someone to help you interpret it and put it into context. For that purpose, consult your low-vision specialist, as well as your GP. The low vision specialist may help you select various optical and other aids that will help you function better in many tasks, including driving.

A list of eye care specialists may be obtained from your state optometric association, the State Commission for the Blind, the

State's Association of the Blind and Visually Impaired and other local agencies. Many other resources for information and referral are listed in Appendix B.

## Know the law and your legal status

Laws and regulations governing driving with low vision change frequently, reflecting the increasing amount of research data, information, and evolving attitudes toward the issue.

Appendices A and E in this book contain information regarding federal and state statutes and regulations concerning driving with low vision and visual screening tests.

As you can see in Appendix A, the federal law prohibits discrimination against persons with low vision conditions, and the official position of the Department of Transportation is that the use of Bioptic telescopes **cannot** be the sole ground for disqualifying someone from driving a vehicle.

It is important to know that even if it may be impossible for you to get an unrestricted license, there may still be the possibility of receiving a restricted license. In many states, you may request a driving test to demonstrate that you can drive safely on a restricted basis.

Before requesting such a test, get evaluated by a driving educator specializing in training people with disabilities (see Appendix B). This way, you can increase your confidence and your chances to pass the test successfully.

Licenses may include the following restrictions:

- Time of day (dawn, dusk, and angle of sunlight)
- Season
- Night driving
- Weather
- Type of road
- Use of specific mirrors and/or other aids
- Accompaniment of a passenger
- Specific roads or areas (of restriction)
- Familiarization with new areas by driving as a passenger each new route

**For specific restricted license options, please refer to Appendix E: State Requirements, and your local DMV.**

⇨ **Remember:** Even if you don't get a full, unrestricted, license, you may still be able to drive with a restricted license!

"I was heartbroken when I was told I could drive only during daylight," said S. B., a bioptic telescope driver who started her driving career in Pennsylvania. "But on the other hand, I was grateful that I could drive at all."

Because rules and regulations change frequently, we recommend that you use the information in this book as a general reference. Before taking any practical steps, contact your local DMV and ask them for their latest position on the relevant subject — in writing.

If you feel that you are not receiving prompt or clear answers to your questions from government authorities, you may want to contact your local representative or senator.

## Know the latest technical developments in low vision

Keep abreast of the latest scientific and technological developments relevant to low vision and driving. Many professionals are working diligently to create new techniques and technologies that may work to your advantage.

Appendix D of this book contains an up-to-date list and descriptions of the most relevant visual aids for low vision driving. Since there are constant developments and changes, we recommend that you keep in touch with your eye specialist. Do not hesitate to contact your local Optometric Association, the American Academy of Ophthalmology, your state DMV and the American Association of Retired Persons (AARP) with questions regarding the current status of technologies and vision care products.

⇨ **Remember:** Driving is a dynamic, ever-evolving activity, requiring a constant level of concentration and the ability to react to both the expected and the unexpected with an equal degree of competence and confidence. Make sure you are ready for this challenge.

## Know who plays a role

As an individual with a low vision condition, when contemplating acting to sustain or reinstate your driving privileges, make sure you receive proper advice, information and training from skilled individuals.

The list below describes professionals whose field of expertise may be relevant to your quest for driver's license.

**Eye Care Specialist** — The eye care specialist (ophthalmologist or optometrist) will most probably be involved in diagnosing your condition and assessing if and what can be done to improve or sustain your vision using medical, surgical and optical approaches, to a point where it may be both legal and safe for you to drive.

**Vision Rehabilitation Specialist** — The vision rehabilitation specialist (ophthalmologist, optometrist, low vision therapist, or occupational therapist specializing in low vision rehabilitation) will participate in setting up a vision rehabilitation and/or training program for you. Such a plan can contribute greatly in preparing you to resume or regain your ability to drive safely, as well as improve your ability to function in other areas.

**Driver Educator** — Learning to drive with a visual disability is no task for amateurs. You have to learn new 'tricks' to compensate for your visual deficiencies, to optimize your visual control of the road and your ability to detect and react to both routine and emergency driving conditions. It is crucial that you undergo training prior to testing for or resuming driving. Make sure that your driving educator is accredited by the state, or by a national organization, to train low vision drivers.

Appendix B, at the end of this book, contains references to various professional organizations that are active in the low vision and driving fields. Please note that inclusion or the exclusion of a certain group or organization in the list does not imply endorsement or recommendation, positive or negative by the authors.

**Note:** In different states, low vision driving professionals may have different titles, such as 'Low Vision Therapist', or 'Orientation and Mobility Instructor'. Please check with your low vision specialists and the local Association for the Visually Impaired for the exact terms and titles in your area.


## MAKING A DECISION

After you satisfy yourself that you have collected and considered all the information that may be relevant to your decision, you may want to sit down and make a checklist similar to the following:

- **Is my health condition (including vision) stable?** Yes / No
- **Has my eye care specialist (or low vision specialist) said I could drive with my condition?** Yes / No
- **Has my General Practitioner said I could drive with my condition?** Yes / No
- **Do the laws and regulations in my state enable me to drive with my condition?** Yes / No

■ **Do I want to go through the steps necessary to acquire/retain a low vision driver's license?** Yes / No

■ **Do I have the financial resources needed to get a license?** Yes / No

If the answer to all the questions above is **Yes**, you are ready to launch a bid for your low vision driver's license. If one or more of the answers is **No**, you probably want to re-evaluate your condition and/or position and solicit additional advice or help from friends and professionals. You may also decide that you should not pursue driving.

The next chapter will take you through the specific steps required to train, acquire the necessary skills and qualify for your low vision driver's license.

# CHAPTER 5
# GETTING READY TO DRIVE

## ACTING ON YOUR DECISION

Having decided to go ahead and get/reclaim/extend your low vision driving license, there are still several things you should do before you can embark on the actual driver's training program. These steps include selecting the best vision aid or aids; learning to use the vision aids effectively without a car, and finally, a search for a suitable and qualified driving instructor.

## Getting the right vision aid(s)

With the aid of the right professional, select the proper vision aid to optimally suit your condition. It may be that you do not need elaborate vision aids, and that simply getting a better spectacles' prescription will enable you to pass the screening test and drive safely. If this is not sufficient, there are a number of other options.

Here are a few examples:

### *Bioptic telescopes*

People with reduced visual acuity and intact peripheral vision use bioptic telescopes. The telescopes are used to read road signs and examine faraway objects.

Investigate the possibility of using a bioptic telescope (in the states that allow them, and in those states that do not explicitly prohibit their use — see Appendix E). Ask to see and try more than one type of bioptic telescope. There are many variations (see Appendix D) and different people prefer different telescopes.

⇨ **Remember:** If you need and can use bioptic telescopes, make sure that your carrier lenses (your regular glasses, on which the telescopes will be mounted) give you the best possible vision. You will be using your carrier lenses most of the time while driving. You will use the bioptic telescopes only for brief periods, for spotting and reading road signs.

There are a number of novel telescopic devices that have not been used for driving yet but may be used for this purpose in the future. Find more about the advantages and limitations of these types of devices in Appendix D.

## Electronic car navigation system

Navigation is a major component of the driving task and requires a share of the driver's mental resources. It is therefore much easier to drive in one's own neighborhood than in a foreign city. Driving navigation involves both finding the correct route and responding in a timely manner to road signs and markings. The recent development of car navigation devices carries a promise to reduce the demand on drivers' resources, and ease the task of finding your way in an unfamiliar setting.

## Peripheral visual field devices

For people with peripheral field loss such as in glaucoma and retinitis pigmentosa (RP) as well as hemianopia, a number of optical devices for field expansion may be available. Most of these devices are aimed at helping patients with very severe field loss, who have difficulty walking. Some of these devices are now being evaluated for driving as well. In particular, devices for patients with hemianopia are being considered as driving visual aids. Additional mirrors are required for driving with field loss in some jurisdictions. Special wide field minifying mirrors are available as well and may be considered as a visual aids for such patients.

**For more detailed information about these and other low vision aids, please refer to Appendix D — Low Vision Driving Aids.**

## Finding a qualified driving instructor

Finding a qualified and suitable driving instructor may not be a simple process. Yet, it is crucial that you take the time to select the professional that you feel most comfortable with, and that you think will maximize your chances to get a driver's license and to drive safely afterward.

For a complete and updated list of certified driver rehabilitation specialists in your state, get in touch with:

The Association for Driver Rehabilitation Specialists (ADED)
P.O. Box 49, Edgerton, WI 53534
Tel: (608) 884-8833
Fax: (608) 884-4851

**Note:** Local associations for the visually impaired and local support groups may also provide referrals to experienced driving instructors.

Rehabilitation hospitals treating stroke patients frequently have a driving rehabilitation program, and may be able to provide a reference.

After you have received the contact numbers of several instructors in your area, do the following:

■ Call each instructor, describe your condition briefly, inquire if the instructor has experience training persons with your condition, and ask for references — preferably from people with your condition or a similar kind of condition.

- Try to get a feel for the character of the instructor. Remember that you will spend a lot of time in the confines of a car together, and some of it may be tense. It is important that you feel comfortable with your instructor and trust his/her judgment.
- Call the references; discuss the instructor's positives and negatives. Be as blunt as you need to be, and try to get straight answers.
- Shop around. Inquire about total cost, and try to determine possible hidden costs.

**Note:** In major metropolitan areas there may be several qualified instructors.

## Getting used to the new vision aid

Having acquired the right vision aid, start a comprehensive training program, with the guidance of a professional, to sharpen the following skills:

- Using the vision aid without driving.
- Using the vision aid on the road (as a <u>passenger</u>).

If your vision screening test results are marginal (you did not pass the screening test, but your results are close to the legal limit), do not give up. Get as much professional training and guidance as possible, and than take a repeat test, this time in a way that will improve your chances of passing.

If you fail the screening test, you can ask for a retest using a chart instead of looking into the screening device used by many DMVs. The increased light and contrast on the chart may be sufficient to make the difference.

Make sure that you get the best possible glasses prescription **before** you request a second test. A small change in the prescription may be all that you need.

In some states, your eye care professional may be able to test you in her/his clinic, and certify to the DMV that you pass the screening test with the new correction. Ask your DMV about this arrangement.

Testing **inside** your eye doctor's office may be less stressful than testing in the DMV office. In some cases, this change alone may enable you to pass the test you may have otherwise failed.

For information regarding repeated vision screenings, please refer to the tables in Appendix E — State Vision Requirements.

Now, everything is ready to start your actual low vision driver's training course! In the next chapter, we will describe a structured training regime that will maximize your skills and safety in learning to use your vision aid on the road.

# CHAPTER 6
# LEARNING TO DRIVE

## A STRUCTURED APPROACH TO LOW VISION DRIVER'S TRAINING

Driver training and proficiency development programs for low vision drivers are particularly important to help low vision drivers function successfully on the road.

To qualify for a license, low-vision drivers MUST demonstrate their ability to perform **all** regular driving-related tasks, such as speed control, merging and maneuvering in traffic, use of mirrors, steering and emergency procedures. In addition, they must show that they are able to compensate for specific visual deficiencies through use of aids and/or through particular behavior (such as extra-defensive driving).

⇨ **Remember:** Driver's training may be a very good idea for people who do not have to use any aids, yet are dealing with vision impairment, which may restrict their license in any way.

## Establish a solid training program

The first step that a good driving instructor will take with you when you start your training should be the construction of a coherent and sensible training program. Such a program will gradually increase your proficiency in using your vision aid and will apply this newly acquired proficiency to the unique circumstances associated with your condition and with low vision driving.

Such a program will probably contain four major parts:

- Learning to use your vision aid
- Training at home
- Training on the road
- Testing

## Learn to use your vision aid

The use of a specific vision aid such as bioptic telescopes requires special training by an experienced professional in a controlled environment.

"I used a bioptic telescope for two years as a passenger, and I was amazed at how little I actually knew about using it properly, until I was shown [how to use it] by a professional instructor," says M. S., a bioptic telescope driver from New Hampshire.

Before you get behind the wheel, it is necessary to receive specific training to learn when and how to properly use the bioptic telescopes:

1. Learn to judge distances of stationary objects (you are stationary).

2. Learn to judge distances of moving objects (you are stationary).
3. Learn to judge distances of moving objects (you are in motion).
4. Visual memory training.

## Training at Home

You can sharpen your control and understanding of your bioptic telescope at home with a series of exercises:

1. **Vertical and Horizontal Sighting and Fixation** — Find a target through the regular spectacle lens (the carrier lens), point your head towards it and try to find it through the telescope as quickly as possible. Look at the target only as long as it is necessary to recognize what it is. Find it again through the carrier lens. Repeat the exercise for targets across the whole field of view.

2. **Tracking** — Find a moving object through the carrier lens. Locate the object with the telescope and track it as it moves. Resume tracking through the carrier lens.

3. **Improving Recall** — After viewing a target through the telescope (see previous steps), resume looking through the carrier lens, and try to describe what you saw or read in the target.

4. **Seeing While in Motion** — Repeat the above exercises while sitting as a passenger in a moving car.

## Training on the Road

After you have practiced properly and acquired sufficient skills to feel confident with your bioptic telescope or other low vision aid, you can apply for a student-driver permit (if you are a new driver) and begin your driver's training.

If you are a licensed driver, you will still need to receive additional training in the specific driving skills associated with low vision from a certified driving educator.

The driver's training period may be about 20 hours, but will vary considerably depending on your skills and level of vision disability.

"It took me about two hours to learn how to use the bioptic telescope properly on the road, and after a training period of about 3 weeks (about 15 hours) I felt confident enough to test and drive," says M. S., a bioptic telescope driver from New Hampshire.

Your actual driving training sessions should include:

1. Road positioning and defensive driving (distance, anticipation).
2. Using bioptic and carrier lenses properly.
3. Responding properly to changing levels of illumination and different driving environments (passage from sun to shade, open road to urban congestion).
4. Using dashboard instruments, inside and outside rear-view mirrors.
5. Managing in heavy traffic.
6. Driving at dusk and at night (if practical and legal).
7. Controlling speed.
8. Driving on different types of roads (rural, residential, etc.).
9. Crossing road obstacles (highway construction, narrow bridges, etc.).
10. Accommodation of emergency vehicles.

11. Accommodation of pedestrians.
12. Using colors and shades.
13. Reducing the effects of vibration.

**Note:** No two low vision driving education programs are exactly the same. Your driving instructor will build a customized training program with you, designed to respond to your condition, and the special circumstances of your driving environment (e.g., topography, climate, and illumination).

Practice until you feel confident of your ability to handle any situation you can imagine. When you are ready, get tested by your department of motor vehicle tester. This way you will clearly establish your qualification to drive safely and legally.

**Partial Sources:** (Jose *et al.*, 1983); (Park *et al.*, 1993); (Vogel, 1991)

### Study for and pass the written tests

Learn for and take all the screening and written tests required to receive a driver's license (for the states that require them).

⇨ **Remember:** All initial and advanced driver's training with bioptic telescopes or any other low vision aid should take place under the supervision of a trained and experienced low-vision instructor and/or a certified driver-education instructor with special training in low vision drivers' instruction.

# CHAPTER 7
# ON THE ROAD —
# DRIVING WITH LOW VISION

## THE REALITIES OF LOW VISION DRIVING

Congratulations! Nobody knows better than you that it is not easy to receive or renew your driving privileges with a low vision condition.

Learning to drive with bioptic telescopes and/or with any other low-vision aid is not simple and requires some skills that may not be required from a driver with normal or near-normal vision.

But getting the license is only half the work and fun. The other, even more important part is to use the driving privilege, and to do it wisely.

Now that you are on the road on your own, you would probably want to put your newly acquired freedom to work immediately, going places and meeting people. This is when it becomes doubly critical that you use the accumulating experience of driving with low vision to your advantage, to sharpen your skills and build on your knowledge and understanding of how your condition and driving can interact successfully.

## Acquiring the habits of good driving

The best way to maximize the learning experience from every trip with your car is to think of every trip as a training session. When getting ready to drive, think of yourself as the vehicle's pilot-in-command. You are responsible for taking all possible steps to ensure a safest ride for your passengers, your vehicle, and others on the road.

When using a low vision driving aid, you will probably want to limit your driving to periods that will not extend beyond half an hour to an hour. Keeping constant vigilance with a low vision aid can be tiring, and since you have to be constantly on the alert, you do not want to stretch your resources to the limit. "I feel comfortable for about an hour. Afterwards, I find it difficult to maintain my concentration," say M. S., a bioptic telescope driver from New Hampshire.

Do not rush anywhere. Take your time before starting your engine. Check and double check your bioptic glasses, the windshield wipers; double check to ensure that your rear- and side-view mirrors are properly installed and positioned to enable the easiest and most comprehensive view possible.

Make sure your glasses are properly positioned and secured, to enable comfortable viewing both through the telescopes and through the carrier lenses.

## The 19 commandments of the safe driver

The following list contains the do's and don'ts that we think will be most relevant to your success as a low vision driver.

There are probably other important guidelines that you have adopted during the process of studying for and using your driving privileges with a low vision condition. The important thing is to genuinely assimilate your experience and others', so the ideas become an integral part of your behavior on the road. Most likely you are already a safe and conscientious driver. Adopting our commandments and yours will only make you an even better one.

1. Drive your car when it is necessary. Always ask yourself: Is this trip necessary? Could I possibly combine several trips into a single one? Do not drive if the weather and visibility conditions are not favorable.

   The line between using your privilege smartly and abusing it to your detriment passes at exactly the same place where your common sense tells you whether to do or not to do something. Always use your common sense.

2. Plan your trip in advance. Review directions and maps and memorize them before entering your car. If it is going to be a long drive, segment it into manageable sections, to avoid fatigue.

   During the trip, constantly monitor your behavior and reactions. If you feel that your road performance is not up to par, stop immediately and consider your condition off the road.

3. If you have the slightest doubt about your ability to handle your driving tasks safely and successfully, **do not** start the engine! If you are already on the road, stop immediately and safely.

4. Before starting your car, make sure your bioptic glasses, windshield, rear- and side-view mirrors are clean and positioned for best vision and comfort.

   A lot of drivers do their pre-drive checks (safety belt, seat adjustment) while on the move. That is bad, no matter whether you are a low vision or a perfect vision driver.

5. Make sure your telescope is adjusted for the best vision possible. Test your telescopes a couple of times on stationary and moving targets to make sure you are getting the best possible results with minimum head movements.

6. Make sure your glasses are positioned properly on your nose to enable viewing from the telescope (upper part) and carrier lenses (lower part).

7. Make sure you are seated high enough in your seat to enable complete and easy viewing all round. This aids in quick changes from telescope to peripheral viewing. Make adjustments before you start the engine, not afterward.

8. Tape 'Page Magnifier' cutouts on the dashboard dials that you find difficult to locate and read. You can, for example, mark the Speedometer with a bright adhesive tape, and the most important legal speed limits with bright arrows. The fuel tank indicator should also be marked, to avoid getting stuck without

fuel. Check your fuel level **before** you start driving, not while you are driving.

9. Make sure your car is always in top mechanical condition. If in doubt, do not drive. Anything that might detract your attention from the road is a potential hazard. Do not add problems you do not need.

10. Always, day and night, use headlights to increase your visibility and to make yourself more visible to others.

11. **Never** drive under the influence of alcohol and/or drugs.

12. Make a conscious decision to concentrate only on your driving. Never allow yourself to be distracted. Remember: momentary inattention is the largest single cause of traffic accidents. Do not use cellular phone while you are driving, not even the type that is mounted in the car and can be used without hands.

13. Use all your senses to assist you while driving (e.g., listen to cars around you). It may be a wise idea not to listen to the radio either, as it may mask important sounds.

14. A positive attitude promotes safer driving. Always be alert, cautious and calm.

15. Never feel pressured at intersections by drivers behind you. Stay calm and patient while analyzing the distance and speed of on-coming cars. Always be ready for the unexpected.

16. Keep your eyes constantly moving, to cover all pertinent areas. Do not stare at traffic signals. Develop good seeing habits. **See**, **Think**, and **Act**. Remember, much of the information required for driving arrives from the eyes.

17. Always maintain a proper distance from the car in front of you. Space and visibility give you the time needed to make decisions on the move.

18. Always keep enough distance to stop, slow and turn. If you feel that a problem is beginning to develop up ahead, immediately start to slow down, in preparation for a stop. Remember that it's better to slightly annoy the drivers behind you by slowing down than to make an emergency stop and surprise everybody around.

19. Since you must see trouble to avoid it, space and visibility are your best protection for safe driving. Look in the distance, and then zero in on the object you wish to see clearly. Keep your eyes on a target two blocks away inside the city and 0.5 mile ahead on the highway. Look for road blockages ahead. Anticipate lane changes and other corrections before you enter an intersection. Avoid situations that are difficult to get out of.

**Partial Source:** American Bioptic Certified Drivers Newsletter Volume VII.

⇨ **Remember:** You are in charge! Learn to be alert and aware, and to react with confidence and skill.

In Chapter 8, we describe what to do if your quest for a low vision driver's license is less than successful, or if your vision or health evolve in such way that it is no longer possible or safe for you to exercise the privileges of a driver's license.

# CHAPTER 8
# IF ALL ELSE FAILS — HOW TO GET WHERE YOU WANT WITHOUT A CAR

## LIVING WITHOUT A CAR

Sometimes, with all the good-intentions, drive and determination, it is impossible to receive or renew a driver's license. Sure, it's unpleasant, but it's not the end of the world.

In this chapter, we will examine some of the alternatives to self-driving and the ways to find and utilize the public transportation resources available in your community.

## Identifying your transportation needs

Before you spend time and resources identifying and lining up alternate transportation sources, it is necessary that you find out exactly what your transportation needs really are.

To ease the process of identifying and classifying your transportation needs, you can use a table similar to the one presented on the next page.

**Transportation Needs Table**

| Route | Frequency | Distance | Priority | Comments |
|---|---|---|---|---|
| | | | | |
| | | | | |
| | | | | |
| | | | | |
| | | | | |
| | | | | |
| | | | | |
| | | | | |
| | | | | |
| | | | | |
| | | | | |
| | | | | |
| | | | | |

- ■ In the **Route** column, indicate the path of the route.
- ■ In the **Frequency** column, indicate how many times a week (month) you need to take this route.
- ■ In the **Distance** column, indicate the mileage of the specified route.
- ■ In the **Priority** column, indicate whether this is a route you can or cannot do without. Use a five-grade scale to indicate need.

## Combining trips and tasks

The key to creating a livable transportation schedule is your ability to do away with unnecessary trips and to create routes that enable you to accomplish as many tasks in as short and as concentrated a distance as possible.

## Finding and utilizing available transportation resources

Nearly every large urban center in the United States has an organization that provides transportation services to people with various handicaps and limitations to mobility. Usually calling city hall and talking to the receptionist will set you on the way.

If you encounter difficulty identifying transportation providers in your area, contact the public transportation agency or company in your area.

In rural areas, public transportation and special services are sometimes less available. In such cases, you can contact your local taxi service provider and try to arrive at some convenient arrangement with them. Promise them your business, and they may become more flexible on the price. Be clear about when you can be flexible about trip time and when you can't.

## Paying for your transportation

If you play your cards well and make the best of the available public transportation resources in your community, chances are you will be able to recreate some of the sense of independence and mobility that self-driving imparted, and maybe even save some money. Remember the cost of car, car maintenance and insurance you are saving when considering the cost of alternative transportation options.

## Scheduling

If you have to think ahead of time about your trips, you will find that you give them a lot more thought, compared to when you could just jump in your car and go anywhere.

This need to plan ahead of time may prove a money-saving habit, since it will almost inevitably reduce the total number of trips you will take, and will allow you to pay less for your overall transportation needs.

## Pooling

The best way to save money on transportation is pooling. This was true when you drove yourself, and it is even more so when you discover that pooling will considerably reduce the cost of your routine taxi trips, such as shopping, and doctor's appointments.

An ad in the local paper will probably get some responses from people in similar situation as yours. Splitting the costs of transportation will enable you to make more and better use of the available services, and its good for socializing too!

You can also call your local city hall to get additional information regarding group trips to the local shopping mall or downtown area. Shopping centers and health centers may have transportation services available as well.

A recently published book, *Finding Wheels: A curriculum for nondrivers with visual impairments for gaining control of transportation needs*, by Anne L. Corn, is available from amazon.com.

A number of information resources for transportation without a car are listed in Appendix B.

# Chapter 9
## Conclusion —
## Daring to Succeed

### Making an Informed Decision

Not surprisingly, driving with low vision, like many other challenges that we face in life is mostly about our will and determination to succeed. True, sometimes the odds are simply too much against us, but most cases lie somewhere in the gray middle, where our drive, skill and determination — or their absence — determine the outcome.

"What is the most important advice you can give people who are considering driving with low vision?" we asked M. B. of Rhode Island, a bioptic telescope driver with 35 years behind the wheel. "Use common sense," she said. "Know where you are going, know yourself and your limits, drive slowly and don't put yourself on the road more than you have to." While this sounds like an excellent advise to all drivers, this is really the essence of successful driving with low vision: Familiarity, self-knowledge, preparation and caution — together they create the environment that will enable you to exercise your driving privileges in the best way.

And to those of us that think that low vision drivers are a cause for worry, here is what M. B. from Rhode Island has to say about other drivers. "I have friends with perfect vision who drive much worse than me, and I am a nervous wreck when I have to take a ride with them."

The one thing you must bring with you when considering driving with low vision is your will to succeed; the will to pit yourself against the odds with the knowledge that you will come out a winner. So with open eyes and a clear mind, go ahead — Dare to Succeed!

# Appendix A
# Federal Legislation

## The Rehabilitation Act

Section 504 of the Rehabilitation Act states, in part, that "No otherwise qualified handicapped individual in the United States... shall, solely by reason of his handicap, be excluded from the participation in, be denied the benefits of, or be subjected to discrimination under any program or activity receiving federal financial assistance."

As beneficiaries of federal financial assistance, state departments of motor vehicles are obliged to abide by this law.

## How is the Law Interpreted?

In a letter to John C. Whitener, O. D. of the American Optometric Association, Rosalind A. Knapp, a United States deputy general counsel for the Department of Transportation (DOT), states that "We have reviewed the medical, legal, and safety issues and agree that the use of bioptic lenses on a person's eyeglasses should not automatically disqualify him or her from being licensed to drive. Specifically, DOT believes that all driver licenses applicants, whether or not they wear bioptic lenses, should be provided the opportunity to take tests of vision, knowledge and driving skills. Failure to pass such tests should prohibit the issuance of a license. However, if the testing officials conclude that the applicant has passed these tests, the state must issue a license, subject to whatever reasonable restrictions on the privilege to drive that it deems necessary."

"DOT believes that this opportunity for individual knowledge, vision and skill tests complies with the requirements of section 504 of the Rehabilitation Act."

In fact, what DOT really does is to acknowledge that people may be licensed to drive with bioptic telescopes — if they pass all the relevant tests.

A class action suit was filed in December 1986 in the US district court in Pennsylvania based on this law. The suit failed to force the department of motor vehicle to permit driving with bioptics. However, the courts did not order other state licensing agencies in the 3rd district to impose such a ban. Thus, the decision was left up to individual states' licensing agencies.

## THE AMERICANS WITH DISABILITIES ACT (ADA), OF 1990

The stated purpose of the Americans with Disabilities Act (ADA), 1990 is:

(1) "To provide a clear and comprehensive national mandate for the elimination of discrimination against individuals with disabilities";

(2) "To provide clear, strong, consistent, enforceable standards addressing discrimination against individuals with disabilities";

(3) "To ensure that the federal government plays a central role in enforcing the standards established in this act on behalf of individuals with disabilities"; and

(4) "To invoke the sweep of congressional authority, including the power to enforce the fourteenth amendment and to regulate commerce, in order to address the major areas of discrimination faced day-to-day by people with disabilities."

The impact of this law on the driving privileges of people with vision disability is not clear yet. Typically, the interpretation of the law takes place in court when one sues. Only if and when people sue to gain driving privileges based on this law in federal courts will such a decision be made.

# APPENDIX B
# INFORMATION/AID SOURCES

As of April 1999, there were 86 certified low vision therapists in the country. They can be contacted through the following address:

**Association for the Education and Rehabilitation of the Blind and Visually Impaired**
P.O. Box 22397,
Alexandria, VA 22304
Tel: (703) 823-9690
Internet Web address: www.aerbvi.org.

If you cannot find the proper agency in your vicinity, you may find such information by contacting the following organization:

**Lighthouse International of New York**
Information number (800) 829-0500, option 2
Or Tel: (212) 821-9200
Internet Web address: http://www.lighthouse.org/

For a complete and updated list of certified driver rehabilitation specialists in your state, get in touch with:

**The Association for Driver Rehabilitation Specialists (ADED)**
P.O. Box 49, Edgerton, WI 53534
Tel: (608) 884-8833
Fax: (608) 884-4851
Internet Web address: http://www.driver-ed.org/

**The American Association of Retired Persons (AARP)** has an extensive array of contacts and services designed to assist adults with low vision conditions.

**AARP General Information**
Tel: (800) 424-3410
Internet Web Address:
http://www.aarp.org/confacts/caregive/transportation.html

The AARP Driving Program may be contacted through the following:

**AARP 55 Alive/Mature Driving**
601 E. St., NW
Washington, DC 20049
Internet Web Address: http://www.aarp.org/55alive/home.html

The following publications are available by the AARP for persons seeking alternative transportation:

- AARP Independent Living Kit – Transportation (D16428)
- Transportation Tip Sheet (D16231)

The following organization and its internet site disseminates a lot of information about driving with bioptic telescopes

**The National Organization for Albinism and Hypopigmentation**
PO Box 959,
East Hampstead, NH 03826-0959
Tel: (800) 473-2310
Tel and Fax: (603) 887-2310
Internet Web address: http://www.albinism.org/driving/


The following Internet web site contains some information and several links to other sites related to driving with low vision:

Internet Web address: http://www.geocities.com/bioptic_driving/


Additional Transportation resources may be found in the following:

**Community Transportation Association of America**
1341 G. St. NW
Suite 600
Washington, DC 20005
Tel: (202) 628-1480
Fax: (202) 737-9197
Transit HotLine: (800) 527-8279

The National Administration on Aging has substantial information resources concerning mobility program for people without cars.

**National Aging Information Center**
330 Independence Ave. SW
Washington, DC 20201
Tel: (202) 619-0724
Fax: (202) 260-1012

For additional information about low vision and related issues (including driving), you can contact:

**The National Association for Visually Handicapped**
**NAVH San Francisco**
3201 Balboa St.
San Francisco, CA 94124
Tel: (415) 221-3201
Fax: (415) 221-8754
Internet Web address: http://www.navh.org/

**NAVH New York**
22 West 21st St.
NY, NY 10010
Tel: (212) 889-3141
Fax: (212) 727-2931

This Internet site contains a list of Low Vision Specialists:

**The Low Vision Gateway**
http://www.lowvision.org/

Another source of low vision information is:

**Low Vision Information Center**
7701 Woodmont Ave.
Suite 302
Bethesda, MD 20814
Tel: (301) 951-4444

Blind and visually impaired advocacy groups and organizations are also a great source of useful information and referrals:

**AMERICAN COUNCIL FOR THE BLIND (ACB)**
1010 Vermont Avenue NW, Suite 1100
Washington, DC 20005
Toll-free tel: (800) 424-8666

**AMERICAN FOUNDATION FOR THE BLIND (AFB)**
11 Penn Plaza, Suite 300
New York, NY 10001
Tel: (800) 232-5463
E-mail: afbinfo@afb.org

**AMERICAN SELF-HELP CLEARINGHOUSE**
St Clares-Riverside Medical Center
Denville, NJ 07834
Tel: (973) 625-7101

**ASSOCIATION FOR MACULAR DISEASES, INC.**
210 East 64th Street
New York NY 10021
Tel: (212) 605-3719

## COUNCIL OF CITIZENS WITH LOW VISION

1850 Washington Avenue
Clearwater, FL 33755-1862
Toll-free tel: (800) 733-2258

## LIONS CLUBS INTERNATIONAL FOUNDATION (LCIF)

LIONS EYE HEALTH PROGRAM (LEHP) AND
SIGHT FIRST PROGRAM
300 22nd Street
Oak Brook, IL 60521
Tel: (630) 571-5466
Web: http://www.lionsclubs.org

## NATIONAL ASSOCIATION FOR PARENTS OF THE VISUALLY IMPAIRED (NAPVI)

PO Box 317
Watertown, MA 02272
Toll-free tel: (800) 562-6265

For the **US Department of Veterans Affairs**, Visual Impairment Services Team and other federal government agencies, see US Government listings in local telephone directory.

The American Optometric Association is also a good source of information regarding Low Vision Specialists:

**American Optometric Association**
Low Vision Section
243 N. Lindbergh Blvd.
St. Louis, MO 63141
Tel: (314) 991-4100, ext. 238

Additionally, the American Optometric Association publishes a list of State Optometric Associations. You can call your local association to receive information about doctors of optometry in your area who specialized in low vision care.

# Appendix C
# Terms You Should Know

## Low Vision

Low Vision is defined as a reduction in the visual capabilities due to disease or injury that impacts the person's ability to perform visual tasks (causing disability). Usually, a person is considered to have low vision when he/she cannot read newspaper-size print with standard spectacle or contact lens correction. In addition, a person with severely reduced peripheral visual field is considered to have low vision even if the visual acuity is maintained, if the reduced field limits the ability to perform tasks such as driving.

## Legal Blindness

In most states and under federal law, legal blindness is defined as having a visual acuity in the better-seeing eye of 20/200 or worse (with the best regular glasses or contact lenses correction). This figure actually means that a person is capable of reading only the big top **E** on the standard eye chart. Legal blindness status is also recognized in cases where there is loss of peripheral visual field — when the visual field in each eye is less than 20 degrees in diameter (tunnel vision).

Still, a person who is legally blind due to visual acuity problems may qualify to legally drive in many states (with the proper visual aid, training, and evaluation).

## LOW VISION AIDS

Low vision aids are devices, either optical, electronic, or others that are used by visually impaired persons to enable them to perform visual functions more effectively. Typically, low vision aids provide magnification or increased contrast. In some cases, they serve to increase the visual field. See Appendix D for more details.

## LOW VISION DRIVER'S TRAINERS

Some driving instructors are specialized and certified to train people with various disabilities. Many of these instructors offer special training to persons with low vision, either due to reduced visual acuity or reduced visual field. In addition to effective use of the visual aids, low vision driver's trainers train their clients in route planning, defensive driving and many other skills necessary for safe operation of car with reduced vision.

## MOBILITY TRAINERS/INSTRUCTORS

Mobility trainers are professionals who teach the severely visually impaired independent mobility techniques. In addition to teaching the use of the long cane to avoid obstacles and increase safety, mobility trainers teach their clients route planning, safe walking and street crossing techniques and effective use of public transportation.

## VISUAL SCREENING TESTS

The vision tests administered at the time of license application and/or renewals by most departments of motor vehicles (DMV) are called visual screening tests. Failing a screening test does not automatically disqualify you from receiving a valid driver's license. It means, in many cases, that you must take additional tests, (vision and/or driving). If successful, in many cases a driver's license may be issued, although it might carry restrictions.

## VALID DRIVER'S LICENSE

It is important to understand that possessing an **un-expired** driver's license does **not** automatically mean that the license is also **valid**. To maintain the validity of a license (in most jurisdictions), the user is obliged to report to the responsible authority every change in his/her health/medical and mental condition, including but not limited to vision problems. If you are driving with an invalid license, your insurance coverage may not be binding.

## RESTRICTED LICENSE

A restricted license is a permit to drive under certain limitations. They may include:

■ Time of day
■ Season
■ Weather Conditions
■ Type of Road

> ⇨ **Remember:** A person who is legally blind due to a visual field restriction may have 20/20 vision in each eye and still NOT be qualified for driving according to regulations in many states.
>
> In fact, a person with such a severe visual field loss should not be driving, even in states that do not have a legal requirement for visual field testing for driving.

## GLARE CONTROL

### Night glare

Glare, especially when driving at night, is one of the most distracting conditions, and a cause of considerable difficulty among drivers with normal and low vision alike. Due to imperfections in the eye's optics (cornea, lens, retina), the bright light from oncoming headlights scatters inside the eye, causing a veil-like translucent obstruction that impedes visibility. Glare and its control may become an even more acute problem for people with cataract (even after cataract surgery), corneal problems, and diabetic retinopathy, because of the increased scatter of light in the effected eyes.

In recent years, a new type of brighter car head light was introduced called HID (High Intensity Discharge). These headlights provide 3 to 4 times more illumination for the driver, and are therefore an advantage to older drivers who need more light to see. However, the HID lights cause more glare problems for oncoming drivers. While many people complain about these new lights, no evidence has been presented to date that they compromise safety on the roads.

The effect of glare may extend even after the glare-causing car has passed. This is an after-effect (after-image) similar to that experienced when exposed to the blinding flash of a camera.

The car's visor may be used to control night glare to some extent, but the help it provides is minimal. Glare from the windshield at night may make night driving a difficult and sometimes unsafe undertaking. This glare can be controlled effectively by maintaining a clean windshield, by using a variety of anti-glare products such as Rain-X, and keeping the windshield wipers in good order.

To combat glare from behind (tailing cars with main or high beams reflected in the rear-view mirror), most cars are equipped with an anti-glare device that tilts the inner part of the rear view mirror at an angle that deflects the glare yet allows viewing of cars behind you. Some recent model cars are equipped with a device that causes the rear view mirror and side mirrors to darken when impacted with high intensity light. If you are in the market for a new car, it may be worth checking with your dealer about the availability of this feature in various models that you are considering. Such mirrors, using electrochromic technology (Chang and Werner, 1999) are distributed by Donnelly Corporation, and it may be possible to find such mirrors that will fit your current vehicle.

Special spectacles, where only the left part of both lenses is tinted dark as in sunglasses, were invented and patented by a number of individuals to provide a useful control of oncoming cars' lights glare. Though the devices are fairly effective and easy to use, we are not aware of any commercial products that offer this design. Possibly these spectacles were never manufactured because of safety concerns relating to the risk of missing a non-illuminated object that falls into the field of the dark lens. One may build such glasses from clip-on sunglasses, but a careful fitting for each individual is needed for proper and safe use. In addition, most clip-on sunglasses may not be dark enough to provide sufficient glare relief.

## Daylight glare (solar glare)

During the day, direct glare from the sun and reflections off the road or off a car's engine hood may be controlled with the aid of sunglasses. Solar glare is particularly disturbing in the winter when the sun is lower in the skies. In addition, window frost can significantly and dangerously increase the effect of solar and night glare.

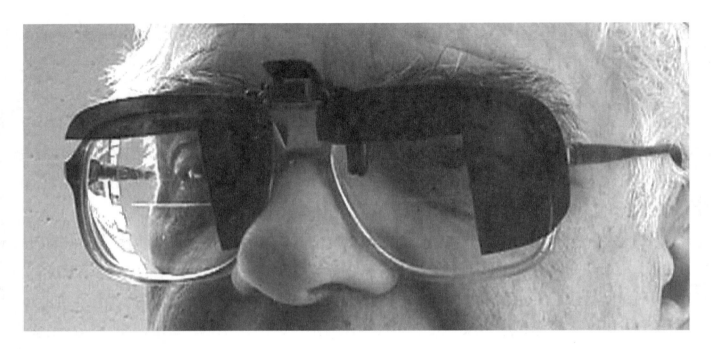

**A homemade glare control clip-on. This device was made by cutting a commercially-available clip-on sunglasses. The residual side sections are used to block headlight glare, while the top strip can be used to block and control solar glare. In all cases, only slight head movements are needed to operate the device.**

It is therefore crucial to completely and thoroughly clean the windshield before getting on the road.

Polarized sunglasses are different from other sunglasses in their ability to selectively block light reflecting from horizontal surfaces such as the road or bodies of water (lakes, rivers). However, they offer no particular protection against direct glare from the sun.

The car's visors may be used to block the direct glare of the sun when it is low on the horizon, such as in the early morning hours and in late afternoon. Many drivers find that the solar glare can impair their vision drastically when it comes in through the space between the visors and the rear view mirror. Recent model cars are frequently equipped with an extension of the visors (fixed or moveable) that can block this space. It may be possible to install such a new visor in an older car or to build a cardboard extension for your existing visor that will do the same thing.

A windshield-cleaning product that effectively reduces glare:

**Rain-X**
c/o Blue Coral - Slick 50 Ltd.
Cleveland, OH 44105

Spray on about once a month. It actually takes much more work than just spraying. The windshield needs to be pre-cleaned, and the product rubbed onto the windshield. But the effect is significant.

⇨ **Remember:** Regular sunglasses are a poor anti-glare solution for night driving. Avoid using sunglasses when driving at night, except for the cutout sunglasses described above.

# APPENDIX D
# LOW VISION DRIVING AIDS

This appendix contains a short description of some of the visual aids available in the market — their use, and their advantages and disadvantages.

If appropriate and legal in your state, a low vision specialist should introduce you to the correct vision aid.

⇨ **Remember: Before** you embark on the road to acquiring a low vision aid, you should get a correct, new prescription for your glasses. This is sometimes overlooked with visually impaired patients.

## BIOPTIC TELESCOPES — TYPES

A bioptic telescope is an optical telescope mounted on the spectacle's lens. The telescope is usually mounted on the upper part of the lens. During normal use, the wearer can look at the environment through the regular spectacle lens (peripheral/carrier lens). When extra magnification is needed, a slight downward tilt of the head brings the object of interest into view through the telescope. The magnified view is used to identify relatively small items, such as road signs and traffic lights. The bioptic telescope can also be used to scan the road ahead, by moving the head from side to side.

Since the field of view visible through the telescope is limited, the telescope should be used only intermittently, and for very short periods — about 1–2 seconds at a time. The field-of-view seen through a spectacle's lenses is very wide and is important for safe driving.

Bioptic telescopes are available with magnification varying from 2.0× to 8.0×. The field of view becomes smaller and consequently the telescope is harder to use with the increase in magnification. Thus, the **smallest** effective magnification should be used. Some states restrict the power of bioptic telescopes that might be used for driving.

Two designs of bioptic telescopes exist, generally known as Galilean and Keplerian:

## Galilean telescopes

The Galilean telescopes are smaller and lighter in weight. Therefore, they are less visible to others and are easier to carry on the nose. This type of optical design is used in so-called "Opera Glasses" which usually have a power of magnification not exceeding 3×. Galilean telescopes have a smaller field of view and usually deliver an image that is less bright than Keplerian telescopes.

## Keplerian Telescopes

The Keplerian telescopes are larger and heavier than Galilean telescopes, but they provide a wider field of view and a brighter image, and are usually easier to use. This is the design typically used in field binoculars.

Both types of telescopes are available with fixed focus or with adjustable focus. For driving, only one level of focus is needed. In general, adjustable-focus telescopes may provide better focusing even for a single focus level, since they allow fine-tuning.

Although telescopes may be used either with one eye or with both eyes, most experts recommend the use of a single telescope for driving. This leaves the field of view of the other eye un-obstructed, even when the telescope is in use, and sidesteps the difficult problem of assuring binocular alignment (i.e. aligning both telescopes so that both eyes are looking at the same point).

## Advantages

The bioptic telescope enables people with visual acuity loss to regain a reasonable degree of visual acuity, sufficient, according to most experts, to safely perform the tasks that are required to drive a car.

The bioptic telescope is allowed and/or accepted as driving visual aid in many states (see tables in Appendix E: State Vision Requirements).

## Disadvantages

The bioptic telescope restricts the visual field when in use. The effect of magnification on perception and apparent motion is difficult to adapt to. Using it effectively and properly requires training.

## BIOPTIC TELESCOPES — BRANDS/MAKES

There are several brands of bioptic telescopes. The following list contains only examples of a few of the many available products and brands. Addresses and phone numbers are provided below. The manufacturers can usually recommend clinicians who can fit their products in various regions of the country, and thus the manufacturers can serve as a referral source.

**Important:** Listing of any of these products here does not constitute a recommendation or an endorsement of the product. It is simply provided as a survey of existing devices. We only have experience fitting patients with some of these devices.

## Designs for Vision Inc.

This is the oldest and most commonly used brand of bioptic telescopes. Numerous models are available with both Galilean and

Keplerian designs. A wide range of powers and designs are available, both fixed and variable-focus.

**Designs for Vision, Inc**
760 Koehler Ave
Ronkonkoma, NY 11779
(516) 585-3300, (800) 345-4009

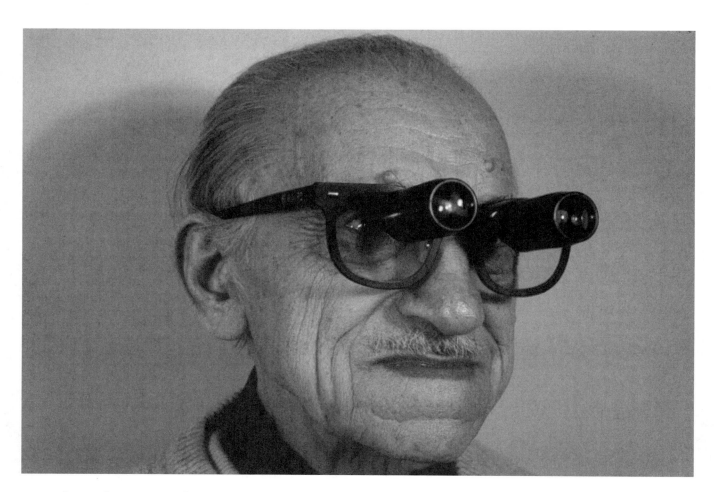

**A patient wearing the binocular Keplerian bioptic telescopes made by Design for Vision, Inc. In most cases only a single (monocular) telescope of this type will be used for driving.**

**(Photo courtesy of Designs for Vision, Inc)**

# BITA® vision enhancer

This is a Galilean micro telescope. It is a very small, hardly noticeable, focusable telescope. It offers a wide selection of powers of magnifications. The small size also supports a perception of simultaneous view of both the magnified and non-magnified views. While simultaneous view may be beneficial as it may permit monitoring the wide field of view when looking at the magnified central view, it may also be confusing. No research was published that addresses these issues.

## Edwards Optical Corporation
P.O. Box 3299
Virginia Beach, VA 23454
(804) 481-4380

# Ocutech Vision Enhancing Systems® (VES™)

This is a periscopic Keplerian bioptic telescope that is mounted across the top of the spectacles rather than sticking out from the lenses themselves. Such a setup is considered more acceptable by many patients. Focusing with these lenses is easier than with most other devices. A recent model even provides for an auto-focus operation similar to that available with auto-focus cameras. This product provides magnifications of 4.0× and 6.0×.

## Ocutech, Incorporated
P.O. Box 625
Chapel Hill, NC 27514
(919) 967-6460 and (800) 326-6460

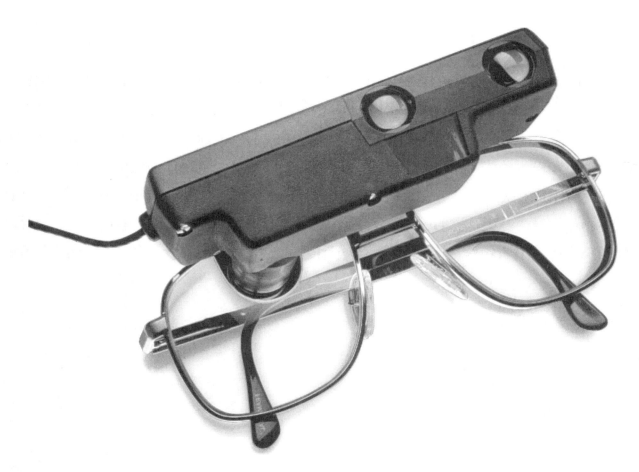

**The VES telescopic system. This system fits over the spectacle frame. Only one eye can be used, but single telescope is preferred for driving. This system is also available with auto focus capability (shown here). The electronic focusing is not necessary for driving and is prohibited in some states.**

**(Photo courtesy of Ocutech, Inc)**

## Behind-the-lens telescope

This is a micro Keplerian system, which is optically folded to fit almost completely behind the spectacle lens. This design is less visible to others. It is also provided in skin-tone for better concealment.

**Optical Designs, Inc.**
1441 Memorial Drive, Suite 13
Houston, TX 77079
(713) 284-8492
Distributor: **Coating Technology Systems, Texas**
800-759-CTSI

**Note:** A number of other low vision device manufacturers have bioptic telescopes available in various designs and powers.

Here are contact details for a few more manufacturers of bioptic telescopes.

**Eschenback Optik of America, Inc.**
904 Ethan Allen Highway
Ridgefield, CT 06877
(877) 422-7300 (Toll Free) and (203) 438-7471
Email: mail@eschenbach-optik.com
www.eschenbach-optik.com

**Keeler Instruments, Inc.**
456 Parkway
Broomall, PA 19008
(800) 523-5620 and (215) 353-4350

## Lighthouse International

Low Vision Products
111 East 59th Street, 12th Floor
New York, NY 10022-1202
(800) 829-0500 and (212) 821-9657
(212) 821-9727 (Fax)
www.lighthouse.org

## Nikon Inc.

1300 Walt Whitman Road
Melville, NY 11747-3064
(800) 645-6687 and (516) 547-4200
(516) 547-0299 (Fax)

## S. Walters, Inc.

30423 Canwood Street, Suite 115
Agoura Hills, CA 91301
(800) 992-5837, (818) 706-2202 and (888) 549-1843
www.walterslowvision.com

## Carl Zeiss Optical Inc.

1015 Commerce Street
Petersburg, VA 23803
(800) 328-2984 and (804) 861-0033
(800) 445-2892 (Fax)

# COMBINED CONTACT LENS/SPECTACLE TELESCOPIC SYSTEMS

The combination of a high, negative-power contact lens and a high, positive-power spectacle lens creates a Galilean telescope, and provide magnification. The level of magnification achieved with such a device is limited and is typically much less than 2.0×.

There are two varieties of the combined contact-lens/spectacle design, one with a single power contact lens and the other with a bifocal contact lens (Filderman, 1959). While such a system may have a slightly wider field-of-view than a similar power bioptic telescope, they significantly restrict the field-of-fixation. The field-of-fixation is that portion of the visual world that the eye could be directed towards using eye movements (Bailey, 1987).

Because of this limitation, it was suggested that this device would be useful only for a patient with minimal need for peripheral vision, or that the best use would be monocular with the other eye used for peripheral vision (Moore, 1964). The field-of-fixation limitation may be a significant drawback for using such a system for driving.

In the bifocal system (Filderman, 1959) the bifocal contact lens is used in conjunction with a bifocal spectacle lens. The carrier lens together with the outer segment of the contact lens are used for peripheral vision with no magnification while the smaller high power inset lens, when combined with the negative power segment of the contact lens, provides magnification with a reduced field. The user can switch at will between the two functions, using eye movement, or head tilt if a special nonconcentric bifocal spectacle lens is used. E. Peli recently applied for a patent for such a system.

Such use may be more suitable for driving, as it is similar to the use of a bioptic telescope. The main advantage of this system over a bioptic is that it is less visible and apparent. The disadvantage is that use of this system requires wearing a hard contact lens that may not be very comfortable. We know of no manufacturer that provides the needed bifocal contact lenses although the special high power bifocal spectacle lenses may be ordered from a variety of sources.

**Note:** We are not aware of any jurisdiction explicitly permitting or prohibiting the use of such systems for driving in the US. The use of these systems, as indeed the use of most other driving visual aids, remains controversial. A few people are known to be driving with such systems in the state of Oklahoma.

## Combined IOL/Spectacle Telescopic System

A telescopic system similar to the combined contact-lens/spectacle system may be constructed using an implanted lens inside the eye, in place of the contact lens. Such lens, called an Intra Ocular Lens (IOL), is implanted in a procedure similar to that used for cataract surgery.

The main advantage of the IOL/spectacle system is that it enables the use of higher magnification (as much as $3.0\times$), and there is no need to wear and care for a contact lens.

There are two varieties of the combined IOL/spectacle design, one with a single power IOL (Choyce, 1964); (Donn and Koester, 1986) and the other with a bifocal IOL (Willis and Portney, 1989); (Koziol *et al.*, 1994). A bifocal IOL/spectacle system developed by Allergan Inc. underwent preliminary testing in the USA several years ago (Koziol *et al.*, 1994). Despite the positive results reported, it has not been brought to market yet.

Optically, these systems are very similar to the combined contact-lens/spectacle system, and they have the same advantages and limitations. There are no reports of anyone using or even recommending these systems for driving, but such use may be attempted if and when they become available commercially.

A similar system is currently under testing in Europe by **Morcher GmbH**.


## Implantable Miniaturized Telescopic (IMT) System

The IMT is a miniature Galilean telescope that is completely implanted inside the eye (Lipshitz *et al.*, 1997); (Peli *et al.*, 2000). The IMT is implanted in place of the crystalline lens and bulges forward through the pupil. The iris is used to support and center the IMT inside the eye near the optical axis.

The IMT is implanted using a procedure similar to cataract extraction. It is implanted in only one eye of patients with macular degeneration in both eyes.

The IMT is constructed from two glass lenses inside a glass tube. Together with the cornea, the IMT acts as a 3.0× magnification telephoto lens that is in focus at a distance of 20 inches. With the use of regular spectacle lenses, the IMT can be focused at any distance.

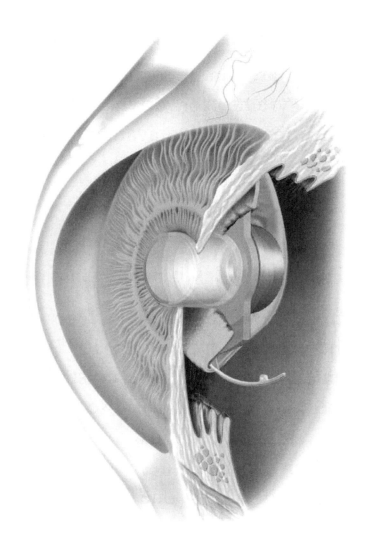

**An illustration of the implantable miniaturized telescope (IMT) that is completely included inside the eye.**

The field-of-view through the telescope is limited to 6.6°. For this reason, the telescope is implanted in one eye only to provide high-resolution vision, while the other eye continues to be used to monitor the wide peripheral field and for safe mobility. While the field-of-view is small, the field-of-fixation, the ability to scan using eye movements, is essentially not limited and thus provides an important advantage over other telescopic systems.

The IMT has been approved for clinical use in Europe since the year 2000. Studies are under way to gain approval in the USA. While it is not specifically designed as a driving aid, it represents a new type of distance vision aid that may be found suitable for driving among other applications.

The IMT is developed and marketed by VisionCare Ltd.

**VisionCare, Ltd.**
3 Moshe Dayan Rd. POB 11373
Yehud
ISRAEL 56101
011-972-632-3055
European Office: 011-41-481-7711

## REVERSED TELESCOPE FOR TUNNEL VISION

Reversed telescopes, designed to minify (make smaller) everything seen through them, were proposed as a vision aid for patients with tunnel vision. The minification increases the instantaneous field-of-view, but at the same time reduces resolution and visual acuity.

This limits the practical minification to less than 2.0 and thus provides for a fairly limited field expansion.

We are not aware of any jurisdiction that explicitly permits the use of such field expansion devices. A few states explicitly prohibit them. However, the expansion provided is unlikely to meet visual field screening requirement in any state that has such requirements, except in cases of minimal field loss.

## Amorphic reversed telescope for tunnel vision

The Amorphic lens developed by Designs for Vision Inc. is a reversed telescope similar to the one described above. The difference is that the Amorphic lens minifies images only in the horizontal dimension and not in the vertical. The result is that everything seen through it looks thin and tall. This provides an expansion of the horizontal field of view and reduces the resolution loss due to the minification.

A recent study (Szlyk *et al.*, 1998) investigated the use of the Amorphic lens mounted in the lower part of the lens (bifocular position), and used intermittently in driving simulation. An improvement was noted with the use of the Amorphic lens and extensive training. Unfortunately, the Amorphic lens has been discontinued and is no longer available. Other reversed telescopic systems are still available from a number of manufacturers of bioptic telescopes.

## *Appendix D*

# HEMIANOPIA VISUAL FIELD DEVICES

For patients with **hemianopia** — the loss of the visual field on one side — other devices are recommended. Typically, either mirrors or prisms are used to expend the field of vision or to increase awareness on the side affected by the loss of field of vision.

In all cases, these devices afford a small change in field of vision. The value of these devices for driving has not been formally evaluated in studies.

While many states do not qualify patients with hemianopia for a driving license by the screening criteria, some patients receive their license after passing a specific driving evaluation. The prism devices may help improve and/or ease performance in such tests. A few states specify that field-testing cannot be performed with the aid of field expansion devices.

## Visual field awareness system

This is a system using prism segments placed within the spectacle lens on the side of the visual loss. This arrangement increases the field by a few degrees when the patient is looking through the prism. However, the increase in field of vision is due to diplopia (double vision) generated by the prism. This diplopia is very bothersome, and patients frequently reject the use of these devices because of what they describe as unacceptable side effects.

**Rekindle**
Gottlieb Vision Group
5462 Memorial Drive, Suite 101
Stone mountain, GA 30083
Tel (Toll Free): (800) 666-7484
Tel: (404) 296-6000

**Field Expanding Lenses (binocular prisms)**

These are molded lenses that include the prism correction in them, mainly for aesthetic reasons. The prism is included in half the lens, and the prescription may be ground into the lens.

The traditional use of prism for both lenses does not increase the field of vision; it only shifts it towards the seeing side when the patient is looking through the prism. The benefit of such correction is limited.

This kind of prism was provided in the past by:

**Inwave Inc.**
Janesville, WI

**Note:** Inwave stopped operations in 1999.

Similar lenses can be obtained from Chadwick Optical.

## Peripheral prism segment on one lens only

Peli (2000) has proposed a new method for correction using a prism segment on one lens only. In this design, the prism segment spans the entire width of the lens, but is limited to the upper and lower peripheral parts of the lens. This enables field expansion when the user looks right or left.

The prism causes peripheral diplopia (see explanation above). However, peripheral diplopia is much easier to adapt to than the central diplopia induced by other methods. The use of stronger prism segments is also possible due to the peripheral location of the segment in this design. A stronger prism in this case means a wider

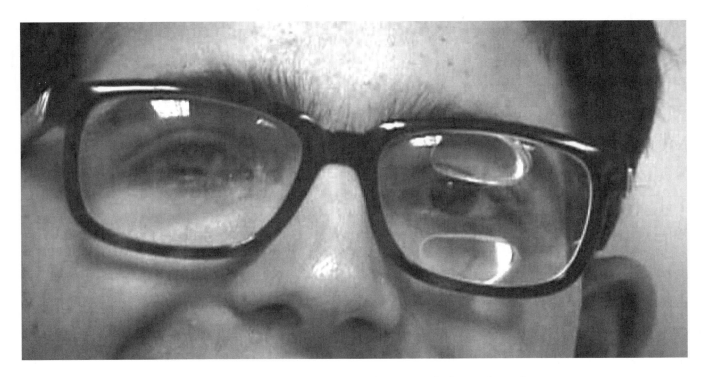

**A patient wearing the spectacles with peripheral prism segments inserted both above and below the pupil.**

expansion of the field. As it is used today, this system provides a visual field expansion of about 20 degrees. That is a significant increase, but on its own may be sufficient only in few cases to provide the span of field required by most state regulations. Special testing and approval will therefore be needed for patients wishing to use this system to regain driving privileges.

Two types of prisms may be used for this device. A press-on prism is manufactured by 3M and is available from most ophthalmic suppliers. These prisms are cut to fit the spectacle frame and are simply pressed onto the spectacle lens. There is a need to replace the lenses every few months as the optical quality and the adhesion to the lens deteriorate.

A permanent plastic prism segment may be mounted into the spectacle lens by MultiLens Inc or by Chadwick Optical Inc:

**MultiLens**
Hönekullavagen 7
BOX 220
MÖLNLYCKE S-435 25
SWEDEN
Tel: +46-31-88-75-50
Website: www.multilens.se/eng/main.asp

**Chadwick Optical Inc**
P.O. Box 485
White River Junction, VT 0501
Tel: (800) 410-1618

## BLIND SPOT MIRRORS

Special mirrors may be installed on the interior and exterior rearview mirrors in the car to provide especially wide field of view. These mirrors, distributed by Brookstone stores across the country, are small minifying mirrors provided with self-adhesive backing to be installed on the car's mirrors. The high level of minification provided by these mirrors results in a very wide field of view. That may be of special value for people with restricted visual fields. A look at such a mirror will provide a wider coverage of the field than is possible with the original car's mirrors. They are meant to compensate for the car's blind spots but may do the same for the person's blind spots. The loss of resolution due to the minification is compensated by the availability of the view with the rest of the original mirror. Of course, with these mirrors the warning regarding objects being closer than they appear is even more relevant.

Brookstone website: http://www.brookstone.com

## ELECTRONIC NAVIGATION DEVICES

Electronic navigation devices using the satellite-based Global Positioning Systems (GPS) are becoming more common every day. A variety of systems are offered with new cars, and many car rental companies offer them as an option, which may be a great way to evaluate the usefulness of such systems. Many of the systems offer help in locating your position and in finding the way back to the main road when you are lost, using two-way communication with a staffed control center. Other systems prompt you to dial in your destination and then provide driving direction by way of maps and even audible directions.

Motorola is developing a new car communication, entertainment and navigation system. The system, called iRadio™, is designed to minimize the time that the eyes have to be off the road and the time that the hands have to be off the wheel for operation. It uses a familiar radio dial design and applies speech output to provide directions and information to the driver, and voice recognition technology for the operator control of the system. In addition to the navigation capability the system provides radio, cell phone, and a variety of selectable information services such as weather and point of interest searches.

In the navigation mode, the system will combine a GPS satellite based technology to follow the car's location with updated road status and traffic information obtained from the internet, using cell phone communications to guide the driver through the best route to his destination. The route can be requested from the car using either the knob controls (with speech output) or with spoken commands. In addition, the route can be pre-planned from home using an Internet website. With this feature the driver can learn and review the planned route and then recall it from the car. While on the road, the system will provide spoken directions including exact turning points and highway exit forewarnings. The effect is similar to having a person who knows the way sitting next to you and giving you directions. In addition, that "person" has constant communication with the traffic control center and knows about road conditions as they are being reported.

While the system has a small screen, as can be seen in the figure below, the display is not intended for use while driving, if at all. The system is designed to be used without taking the eyes off the road, which makes it especially appropriate for use by low vision drivers. Of course the benefits of the system are certainly not limited to that population.

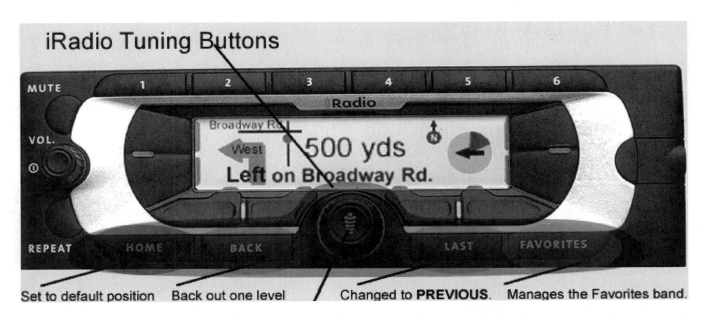

iRadio Tuning Buttons

MUTE  1  2  3  4  5  6

iRadio

Broadway Rd.
West 500 yds
Left on Broadway Rd.

VOL.

REPEAT  HOME  BACK  LAST  FAVORITES

Set to default position  Back out one level  Changed to **PREVIOUS**.  Manages the Favorites band.

**The Motorola iRadio car navigation system provides spoken road direction and cuts down the need to read road and street signs.**

# APPENDIX E
# STATE VISION REQUIREMENTS

## STATE REGULATIONS

This Appendix contains tabulated Visual Screening requirements, methods, and policy information received from Departments of Motor Vehicles across the nation.

⇨ **Remember:** The information in this Appendix is provided as a reference only, and with the understanding that statutes, regulations and attitudes may and will change with time. To receive official, up-do-date information, please contact your local DMV or your low-vision specialist.

## States Permitting Bioptics

The following states officially allow the use of bioptic telescopes for driving:

| | | |
|---|---|---|
| Arkansas | Massachusetts | Oregon |
| California | Michigan | Pennsylvania |
| Colorado | Mississippi | Rhode Island |
| Delaware | Missouri | South Carolina |
| Georgia | Montana | South Dakota |
| Idaho | Nebraska | Tennessee |
| Illinois | Nevada | Texas |
| Indiana | New Hampshire | Vermont |
| Kansas | New Jersey | Virginia |
| Kentucky | New York | Washington |
| Maryland | North Dakota | Wyoming |
| | Ohio | |

## States NOT allowing restricted licenses

| | | |
|---|---|---|
| Arkansas | Rhode Island | West Virginia |

## States testing color vision

| Alabama | Massachusetts | Tennessee (Commercial only) |
|---|---|---|
| Arizona (Commercial only) | Montana (Commercial only) | Texas |
| District of Columbia | Nebraska (Commercial only) | Utah (Commercial only) |
| Hawaii | New Jersey | Washington |
| Indiana (Commercial and bioptic only) | North Carolina (Commercial only) | Wisconsin (Commercial only) |
| Kentucky | North Dakota (Commercial only) | |
| Maryland (Commercial only) | Ohio (Commercial only) | |

## States testing visual field

| Alabama | Maryland | Oklahoma |
|---|---|---|
| Arizona | Massachusetts | Oregon |
| Arkansas | Michigan | Pennsylvania |
| Connecticut | Minnesota | Tennessee |
| District of Columbia | Missouri | Utah |

| | | |
|---|---|---|
| Florida | Montana (Commercial only) | Vermont |
| Georgia | Nebraska | Virginia |
| Hawaii | Nevada | Washington |
| Illinois | New Mexico (if failed screening) | Wisconsin |
| Indiana | New York | Wyoming |
| Iowa | North Carolina (Commercial only) | |
| Kentucky | North Dakota | |
| Maine | Ohio | |

**Note:** While many of these states officially test for visual field, the tests are frequently omitted or are ineffective.

## States testing depth perception

| | | |
|---|---|---|
| Colorado | Hawaii | N. Dakota |
| Connecticut | Kentucky | Utah |

## States testing eye coordination

| | | |
|---|---|---|
| Colorado | Hawaii | N. Dakota |

## States testing luminance contrast

No State

## States allowing qualified drivers to drive at night with bioptic telescopes

In some of these states, there is no official policy against driving at night, and no explicit permission.

| Carolina | New York | Tennessee |
|----------|----------|-----------|
| Colorado | Ohio | Virginia |
| Georgia | Oregon | Wyoming |
| Michigan | South Carolina | |

**Sources:** DMV responses to authors' questionnaire, 1997, and updated in 2001; The National Organization for Albinism and Hypo pigmentation website: www.albinism.org

## States in which physicians are required to report a physical/mental disability

| California | Nevada | Texas |
|------------|--------|-------|
| Delaware | North Dakota | |

## States in which physician's report is NOT confidential

| Louisiana |
|-----------|

## States in which license can be suspended upon report from a doctor

| California | Maryland | South Carolina |
|-----------|----------|----------------|
| Delaware | Minnesota | Utah |
| Idaho | New Jersey | Virginia |
| Illinois | New York | Wisconsin |
| Iowa | Oregon | |

Source: (Karmel, 2000)

**Note:** Not all states provided information for the three tables above.

# Tables of state by state vision standards for drivers

**Note:** If your state requirements are not clear from the table, ask your eye specialist.

## Alabama

| License Renewal Procedures | |
|---|---|
| Renewal Interval | 4 Years |
| Vision Screening required | New Drivers |
| Renewal Format | In-Person |
| **Visual Acuity Requirements** | |
| Each Eye Without Correction | 20/40 |
| Both Eyes Without Correction | 20/40 |
| Each Eye With Correction | 20/40 |
| Both Eyes With Correction | 20/40 |
| If One Blind Eye – The other W/O Correction | 20/40 |
| If One Blind Eye – The other With Correction | 20/40 |
| *Absolute Visual Acuity Minimum* | **20/60** |
| **Visual Field Requirement** | |
| **Each Eye / Both Eyes** | N/A / 110° |
| Visual Field Test Method | Keystone View[†] |

| Color Vision Requirement | New and Professional drivers |
|---|---|
| **Allow Restricted License** | Yes |
| Restrictions | Daytime only; Radius restriction[*] |
| **Allow retesting if applicant fails first screening** | Yes |
| Conditions | Vision screening by Eye Care Specialist |
| **Allow Bioptic Telescopes** | No |
| Offer Low Vision Driver's Training / Education | No |

[*]**Radius Restriction:** Driver may not operate the vehicle beyond a specified distance (in miles) from residence.

[†]**Eye Testing Machine**

128

# Alaska

| License Renewal Procedures | |
|---|---|
| Renewal Interval | 5 Years |
| Vision Screening Required | New Drivers / Renewals |
| Renewal Format | In-Person |
| **Visual Acuity Requirements** | |
| Each Eye – Without Correction | 20/40 |
| Both Eyes Without Correction | 20/40 |
| Each Eye With Correction | 20/40 |
| Both Eyes With Correction | 20/40 |
| If One Blind Eye – The other W/O Correction | 20/40 |
| If One Blind Eye – The other With Correction | 20/40 |
| *Absolute Visual Acuity Minimum* | **20/100** |
| **Visual Field Requirement** | No |

| Color Vision Requirement | No |
|---|---|
| **Allow Restricted License** | Yes |
| Restrictions | Daytime; Vehicle type; Specific area; Speed; Others |
| **Allow Retesting If Driver Fails First Screening** | Yes |
| Conditions | Visual Screening by Eye Care Specialist |
| **Allow Bioptic Telescopes** | No |
| Offer Low Vision Driver's Training / Education | No |

# Arizona

| License Renewal Procedures | |
|---|---|
| Renewal Intervals | 12 Years<br>5 Years at age 60+ |
| Vision Screening Required | New Drivers / Renewals |
| Renewal Format | In-Person |
| **Visual Acuity Requirements** | |
| Each Eye – Without Correction | 20/40 |
| Both Eyes Without Correction | 20/40 |
| Each Eye With Correction | 20/40 |
| Both Eyes With Correction | 20/40 |
| If One Blind Eye – The other W/O Correction | 20/40 |
| If One Blind Eye – The other With Correction | 20/40 |
| *Absolute Visual Acuity Minimum* | **20/60** (Both eyes – Daylight driving only) |
| **Visual Field Requirement** | |
| Each Eye | 70°, 35° Nasal |
| Visual Field Test Method | Keystone View[†] |

| Color Vision Requirement | Professional drivers only |
|---|---|
| **Allow Restricted License** | Yes |
| Restrictions | Daylight only |
| **Allow Retesting If Driver Fails First Screening** | Yes |
| Conditions | None |
| **Allow Bioptic Telescopes** | No |
| Offer Low Vision Driver's Training / Education | No |

[†]**Eye Testing Machine**

# Arkansas

| License Renewal Procedures | |
|---|---|
| Renewal Interval | 4 Years |
| Vision Screening Required | New Drivers / Renewals |
| Renewal Format | In-Person |
| **Visual Acuity Requirements** | |
| Each Eye – Without Correction | 20/40 |
| Both Eyes Without Correction | 20/40 |
| Each Eye With Correction | 20/50 |
| Both Eyes With Correction | 20/50 |
| If One Blind Eye – The other W/O Correction | 20/40 |
| If One Blind Eye – The other With Correction | 20/50 |
| *Absolute Visual Acuity Minimum* | **20/50** |
| **Visual Field Requirement** | |
| Each Eye / Both Eyes | 70° / 140° |
| Visual Field Test Method | OPTEC[†] Screening Machine |

| Color Vision Requirement | No |
|---|---|
| **Allow Restricted License** | No |
| **Allow Retesting If Driver Fails First Screening** | Yes |
| **Allow Bioptic Telescopes** | Yes |
| Restrictions | Case by case |
| Absolute Corrected Minimum Through Telescope(s) | 20/50 |
| Absolute Corrected Minimum Through Carrier Lens | 20/50 |
| Require Special Bioptic Telescope Training / Test | No |
| Offer Low Vision Driver's Training / Education | No |

[†]**Eye Testing Machine**

131

# California

| License Renewal Procedures | |
|---|---|
| Renewal Intervals | 5–15 Years |
| Conditions | Driver's qualification for Mail-in renewal |
| Mandatory In-Person Renewal | After age 70 |
| Mandatory Vision Test | Original, upon in-person renewal |
| **Visual Acuity Requirements** | |
| Each Eye Without Correction | N/A |
| Both Eyes Without Correction | N/A |
| Each Eye With Correction | 20/40 |
| Both Eyes With Correction | 20/40 |
| If One Blind Eye – The other W/O Correction | 20/40 |
| If One Blind Eye – The other With Correction | 20/40 |
| *Absolute Visual Acuity Minimum* | **20/200** |
| **Visual Field Requirement** | No |

| Color Vision Requirement | No |
|---|---|
| **Allow Restricted License** | Yes |
| Conditions | Restrictions may vary according to driver's condition |
| **Allow Retesting If Driver Fails First Screening** | Yes |
| Conditions | None |
| **Allow Bioptic Telescopes** | Yes |
| Restrictions | Day only; Periodic retesting |
| Absolute Corrected Minimum Through Telescope(s) | N/A |
| Absolute Corrected Minimum Through Carrier Lens | 20/200 |
| Require Special Bioptic Telescope Training / Test | No |
| Offer Low Vision Driver's Training / Education | No |

# Colorado

| License Renewal Procedures | |
|---|---|
| Renewal Interval | 10 Years after age 21 |
| Mandatory Vision Test | New / Each In-Person renewal |
| **Visual Acuity Requirements** | |
| Both Eyes Without Correction | 20/40 |
| Both Eyes With Correction | 20/40 |
| If One Blind Eye – The other W/O Correction | 20/40 |
| If One Blind Eye – The other With Correction | 20/40 |
| *Absolute Visual Acuity Minimum* | **20/40** Unless approved by Doctor |
| **Visual Field Requirement** | No |

| Color Vision Requirement | No |
|---|---|
| **Allow Restricted License** | Yes |
| Conditions | Daytime; Speed limit 35 mph max; Area: 15 miles radius – are examples based on Doctor's recommendations |
| **Allow Retesting if driver fails first screening** | Yes |
| Conditions | Retest done by a Doctor |
| **Allow Bioptic Telescopes** | Yes |
| Restrictions | Doctor's specified reevaluation. "Tele Lens" appears on license. |
| Absolute Corrected Minimum Through Telescope(s) | N/A |
| Absolute Corrected Minimum Through Carrier Lens | N/A |
| Require Special Bioptic Telescope Training / Test | No |
| Offer Low Vision Driver's Training / Education | No |

# Connecticut

| License Renewal Procedures | |
|---|---|
| Renewal Intervals | 4 Years<br>2 Years after 65 |
| Renewal Format | Every other renewal In-Person |
| Mandatory Vision Test | Every other renewal |
| Vision Screening Required | New drivers |

| Visual Acuity Requirements | |
|---|---|
| Both Eyes With or Without Correction | 20/40 |
| One Blind Eye – The other With or Without Correction | 20/30 |
| *Absolute Visual Acuity Minimum* | Better than **20/200** |

| Visual Field Requirement | |
|---|---|
| Each Eye / Both Eyes | 70° / 100° |
| Visual Field Test Equipment | Optec 1000[†] |

| Color Vision Requirement | No |
|---|---|
| **Allow Restricted License** | Yes |
| Conditions | Daytime only, if vision is better than 20/70 and field of vision is more than 100°. Other restrictions may apply if vision is between 20/70 and 20/200. |
| **Allow Bioptic Telescopes** | No |
| Offer Low Vision Driver's Education | Yes – Graduated Driver's License Program |

[†]**Eye Testing Machine**

# Delaware

| License Renewal Procedures | |
|---|---|
| Renewal Interval | 5 Years |
| Vision Screening Required | New Drivers / Renewals |
| Renewal Format | In-Person |
| **Visual Acuity Requirements** | |
| Each Eye Without Correction | 20/40 |
| Both Eyes Without Correction | 20/40 |
| Each Eye With Correction | 20/40 |
| Both Eyes With Correction | 20/40 |
| If One Blind Eye – The other W/O Correction | 20/40 |
| If One Blind Eye – The other With Correction | 20/40 |
| *Absolute Visual Acuity Minimum* | **20/50 daylight only** |
| **Visual Field Requirement** | No |

| Color Vision Requirement | No |
|---|---|
| **Allow Restricted License** | Yes |
| **Allow Retesting if Applicant Falils First Screening?** | Yes – to be performed by an Eye Care Specialist |
| Conditions | Daytime only |
| **Allow Bioptic Telescopes** | Yes[*] |
| Restrictions | Daytime only |
| Absolute Corrected Minimum Through Telescope(s) | N/A |
| Absolute Corrected Minimum Through Carrier Lens | N/A |
| Require Special Bioptic Telescope Training / Test | Training |
| Offer Low Vision Driver's Training / Education | No |

[*]Low Vision and Bioptic Telescope users are reviewed on a case by case basis by the Medical Advisory Board

# District of Columbia

| License Renewal Procedures | |
|---|---|
| Renewal Interval | 5 Years |
| Vision Screening Required | New Drivers / Renewals |
| Medical Certificate Required | After 70 Reaction Test after 75[*] |
| **Visual Acuity Requirements** | |
| Best Eye Without Correction | 20/40 |
| Other Eye Without Correction | 20/70 |
| Best Eye With Correction | 20/40 |
| Other Eye With Correction | 20/70 |
| If One Blind Eye – The other W/O Correction | 20/40 |
| If One Blind Eye – The other With Correction | 20/40 |
| *Absolute Visual Acuity Minimum* | **20/70** |
| **Visual Field Requirement** | Eye Doctor's report required if only one eye functions |
| Both Eyes | 130° (If less than 130° but more than 110°, may be approved by Director) |
| Testing Method | Confrontation or Perimetry (Binocular) |

| | |
|---|---|
| **Dynamic Acuity Test** | No |
| **Color Vision Requirement** | New Drivers |
| **Allow Restricted License** | Yes |
| Conditions | Acuity not less than 20/70 and daytime, if field of vision is 140° |
| **Allow Bioptic Telescopes** | No |
| Offer Low Vision Driver's Training / Education | No |

[*]Annual eye report for applicant being treated for glaucoma or cataracts unless ophthalmologist indicates other need, or 3 consecutive reports reveal no appreciable deterioration

# Florida

| License Renewal Procedures | |
|---|---|
| Renewal Interval | 6 Years (4 Years if record unclean) |
| Vision Screening Required | New Drivers / Renewals |
| Renewal Format | Mail-In / In-Person every third renewal |
| **Visual Acuity Requirements** | |
| Each Eye Without Correction | 20/50–20/70* |
| Both Eyes Without Correction | 20/50–20/70* |
| Either Eye With Correction | 20/50–20/70* |
| Better Eye With or Without Correction | 20/50–20/70* |
| If One Blind Eye – The other With Correction | 20/40 |
| *Absolute Visual Acuity Minimum* | **20/70** (20/40 if one eye is blind or 20/200) |
| **Visual Field Requirement** | New drivers; renewals; professionals |
| Method of Testing | Normal careful confrontation or Kinetic Perimetry |
| Both Eyes | 130° |

| | |
|---|---|
| **Color Vision Requirement** | No |
| **Allow Restricted License** | Yes |
| Conditions | Daylight driving only |
| **Allow Retesting if Driver Fails First Screening** | Yes |
| **Allow Bioptic Telescopes** | No |

*Below 20/50 requires eye exam.  If vision cannot improve may pass with 20/70

# Georgia

| License Renewal Procedures | |
|---|---|
| Renewal Interval | 4 Years |
| Vision Screening Required | New Drivers / Renewals |
| Renewal Format | In-Person |
| Mandatory Vision Test | Each Renewal |
| Visual Acuity Requirements | |
| Each Eye Without Correction | 20/60 |
| Both Eyes Without Correction | N/A |
| Either Eye With Correction | 20/60 |
| Better Eye With or Without Correction | 20/60 |
| If One Blind Eye – The other With Correction | 20/60 |
| *Absolute Visual Acuity Minimum* | **20/60** |
| Visual Field Requirement | |
| Each Eye / Both Eyes | 140° / 140° |
| Visual Field Testing Method | Juno Vision[†] Machine |

| | |
|---|---|
| **Color Vision Requirement** | No |
| **Allow Restricted License** | Yes |
| Conditions | Daytime |
| **Allow Retesting if Driver Fails First Screening** | Yes |
| Conditions | None |
| **Allow Bioptic Telescopes** | Yes |
| Restrictions | Bi-annual retest |
| Absolute Corrected Minimum Through Telescope(s) | 20/60 |
| Absolute Corrected Minimum Through Carrier Lens | 20/60 |
| Require Special Bioptic Telescope Training / Test | Yes / Yes |
| Offer Low Vision Driver's Training / Education | Yes |

[†]**Eye Testing Machine**

138

# Hawaii

| License Renewal Procedures | |
|---|---|
| Renewal Intervals | 2 Years – Age 72+<br>4 Years – Age 16–17<br>6 Years – Age 18–71 |
| Vision Screening Required | New Drivers /<br>Renewals / Duplicates |
| Renewal Format | In-Person |
| Mandatory Vision Test | Each Renewal /<br>Duplicates |
| **Visual Acuity Requirements** | |
| Each Eye Without Correction | 20/40 |
| Both Eyes Without Correction | 20/40 |
| Each Eye With Correction | 20/40 |
| Both Eyes With Correction | 20/40 |
| One Blind Eye – The other Without Correction | 20/40 |
| If One Blind Eye – The other With Correction | 20/40 |
| *Absolute Visual Acuity Minimum* | **20/40** |
| **Visual Field Requirement** | |
| Each Eye / Both Eyes | 70° / 140° |
| Visual Field Testing Method | Eye Testing Machine, or eye specialist certification |

| | |
|---|---|
| **Color Vision Requirement** | Yes |
| **Allow Restricted License** | Yes |
| **Allow Retesting if Driver Fails First Screening** | Yes |
| Conditions | See Eye Specialist |
| **Allow Bioptic Telescopes** | No |

# Idaho

| License Renewal Procedures | |
|---|---|
| Renewal Interval | 4 Years |
| Vision Screening Required | New Drivers / Renewals* |
| Renewal Format | After 69 In-Person |
| Mandatory Vision Test | Each Renewal Annual if VA < 20/40 |
| **Visual Acuity Requirements** | |
| If One Blind Eye – The other With Correction | 20/40 |
| If One Blind Eye – The other With Correction | 20/50 to 20/60 |
| **Conditions** | Annual Visual and Road Test |
| *Absolute Visual Acuity Minimum* | **Better than 20/70** |
| **Visual Field Requirement** | No |

| Color Vision Requirement | No |
|---|---|
| **Allow Restricted License** | Yes |
| Conditions | Daytime; No Freeways; 5-mile radius from home, In town |
| **Allow Retesting if Driver Fails First Screening** | Yes |
| Conditions | Submit exam results by a vision specialist |
| **Allow Bioptic Telescopes** | Yes |
| Restrictions | Daylight only; Annual visual and road test |
| Absolute Corrected Minimum Through Telescope(s) | 20/40 |
| Absolute Corrected Minimum Through Carrier Lens | 20/60 |
| Require Special Bioptic Telescope Training / Test | No |
| Offer Low Vision Driver's Training / Education | No |

# Illinois

| License Renewal Procedures | |
|---|---|
| Renewal Intervals | 1 year – Age 87+<br>2 years – Age 81–86<br>4 years – Age 21–80 |
| Vision Screening Required | New Drivers |
| Renewal Format | Mail-in |
| Mandatory Vision & Road Test after age | 75 |
| **Visual Acuity Requirements** | |
| Both Eyes With Correction | 20/40 |
| If One Blind Eye – The other With Correction | 20/40 |
| Restrictions | 20/41 – 20/70 Daytime only |
| *Absolute Visual Acuity Minimum* | **20/70** |
| Restrictions | If one eye less than 20/100 – require right and left outside rearview mirrors |
| **Visual Field Requirement** | |
| One eye / two eyes | 105°* / 140° |
| Visual Field Testing Method | Stereo Optical testing machine |

| Color Vision Requirement | No |
|---|---|
| **Allow Restricted License** | Yes |
| Conditions | Daytime; Two outside mirrors |
| **Allow Retesting if Driver Fails First Screening** | Yes |
| Conditions | None |
| **Allow Bioptic Telescopes** | Yes |
| **Restrictions**: Daylight only; No more than 3× wide angle or 2.2× standard. Left/Right outside rearview mirrors (see Visual Acuity Restriction) | |
| Absolute Corrected Minimum Through Telescope(s) | 20/40 |
| Absolute Corrected Minimum Through Carrier Lens | 20/100 |
| Require Special Bioptic Telescope Training / Test | Yes |
| Offer Low Vision Driver's Training / Education | No |

*One eye with 70° temporal field and 35° nasal field qualifies with 2 outside mirrors

# Indiana

| License Renewal Procedures | | | Color Vision Requirement | Yes (for Commercial and bioptic drivers) |
|---|---|---|---|---|
| Renewal Intervals | 4 Years<br>3 Years after age 75 | | **Allow Restricted License** | Yes |
| Vision Screening Required | New Drivers / Renewals | | Conditions | Daytime; Rear view mirror |
| Renewal Format | In-Person | | **Allow Retesting if Driver Fails First Screening** | Yes |
| **Visual Acuity Requirements (see below)** | | | | |
| *Absolute Visual Acuity Minimum* | **20/70** in both eyes | | Conditions | Vision Form by a specialist |
| **Visual Field Requirement** | | | **Allow Bioptic Telescopes** | Yes |
| Each Eye / Both Eyes | 70° / 120° | | Conditions | 4.0× or less<br>20/40 through telescope<br>20/200 through carrier<br>120° field |

| | Color Vision Requirement | Yes (for Commercial and bioptic drivers) |
|---|---|---|

| One eye 20/40 or better, other eye 20/40 or better – No Restrictions |
|---|
| Best eye 20/40 or better, other eye 20/50 to Blind, – Outside rear view mirrors |
| One eye 20/50 or better, other eye 20/50 or better – Glasses Required |
| Best eye 20/50 or better, other eye 20/70 to Blind, – Outside rear view mirror; Daylight Driving only |
| One eye 20/70 or better, other eye 20/70 or better – Outside rear view mirror; Daylight Driving only; Proof of normal peripheral visual fields. |

| Restriction: | Annual vision screening; Annual driving test; Daylight; others as necessary |
|---|---|
| Require Special Bioptic Telescope Training / Test | Yes, min. 30 hours / Extended Test |
| Offer Low Vision Driver's Training / Education | Yes, BMV approved bioptic driver rehab program |

# Iowa

| License Renewal Procedures | |
|---|---|
| Renewal Intervals | 4 Years<br>2 Years if vision is less than 20/40 |
| Vision Screening Required | New Drivers / Renewals |
| Renewal Format | In-Person |

| Visual Acuity Requirements – Unrestricted | |
|---|---|
| Without Correction – Each Eye | 20/40 |
| Without Correction – Both Eyes | 20/40 |
| With Correction – Each Eye | 20/40 |
| With Correction – Both Eyes | 20/40 |
| With Blind Eye – The other W/O Correction | 20/40 |
| With Blind Eye – The other With Correction | 20/40 |

| Restrictions | |
|---|---|

20/50 – Daylight only
20/70 – Restricted Speed – 35mph
20/100 – Discretionary with written recommendation of vision specialist
<20/100 – Requires recommendations of medical advisory board

| *Absolute Visual Acuity Minimum* | **20/200** |
|---|---|

| Visual Field Requirements | |
|---|---|
| Unrestricted | Binocular field 140° |
| Use of L&R outside mirrors | Binocular 115°<br>One eye 70°T + 45°N |
| Advisory board recommendation required | Binocular field <95°<br>Mono. field <60°T+35°N |
| Absolute Minimum of Field | Case by case decision of the board* |
| **Color Vision Requirement** | No |
| **Allow Restricted License** | Yes |

Restrictions: No driving when headlights required, including seasons and variations in weather. Not over 35mph (no highway driving). 20/100 in both eyes – use outside rear view mirrors

| **Allow Retesting If Driver Fails First Screening** | Yes |
|---|---|
| Conditions | Requires a hearing process.<br>May use Doctor's report |
| **Allow Bioptic Telescopes** | No |
| Offer Low Vision Driver's Training / Education | No |

*Lowest approved: 59°

# Kansas

| License Renewal Procedures | |
|---|---|
| Renewal Intervals | 4 Years (16–20, 65+) 6 Years (21–64) |
| Vision Screening Required | New Drivers / Renewals |
| Renewal Format | In-Person |
| **Visual Acuity Requirements** | |
| Each Eye Without Correction | 20/40 |
| Both Eyes Without Correction | 20/40 |
| Each Eye With Correction | 20/40 |
| Both Eyes With Correction | 20/40 |
| If One Blind Eye – The other W/O Correction | 20/40 |
| If One Blind Eye – The other With Correction | 20/40 |
| *Absolute Visual Acuity Minimum* | **No** – Medical Review Board Determines |
| **Visual Field Requirement** | No |

| | |
|---|---|
| **Color Vision Requirement** | No |
| **Allow Restricted License** | Yes |
| Conditions | Daytime only; Distance from Home; No Freeway – Determined by Medical Board |
| **Allow Retesting** | Yes |
| Conditions | None |
| **Allow Bioptic Telescopes** | Yes |
| Restrictions | Daytime only, Annual Vision Screening |
| Absolute Corrected Minimum Through Telescope(s) | N/A |
| Absolute Corrected Minimum Through Carrier Lens | N/A |
| Require Special Bioptic Telescope Training / Test | No |
| Offer Low Vision Driver's Training / Education | No |

# Kentucky

| License Renewal Procedures | |
|---|---|
| Renewal Interval | 4 Years |
| Vision Screening Required | New Drivers / Renewals |
| Renewal Format | In-Person |
| **Visual Acuity Requirements** | |
| Each Eye Without Correction | 20/60 |
| Both Eyes Without Correction | 20/60 |
| Each Eye With Correction | 20/60 |
| Both Eyes With Correction | 20/60 |
| If One Blind Eye – The other W/O Correction | 20/60 |
| If One Blind Eye – The other With Correction | 20/60 |
| *Absolute Visual Acuity Minimum* | **20/80** |
| **Visual Field Requirement** | |
| Each eye | 35° left/right of fixation 25° above/below fixation |
| Visual Field Testing Method | Humphrey, Goldmann III 4e |

| Color Vision Requirement | Yes (new/renewal) |
|---|---|
| **Allow Restricted License** | Yes |
| Conditions | Daytime only |
| **Allow Retesting if driver fails screening** | Yes |
| Conditions | None |
| **Allow Bioptic Telescopes** | Yes |
| Offer Low Vision Driver's Training / Education | Yes |
| Conditions | Visual status stable Horizontal field ≥ 120° Vertical field ≥ 80° |
| Absolute Corrected Minimum Through Telescope(s) | 20/60 |
| Absolute Corrected Minimum Through Carrier Lens | 20/200 |
| Require Special Bioptic Telescope Training / Testing | Yes / Yes |

# Louisiana

| License Renewal Procedures | |
|---|---|
| Renewal Interval | 4 Years |
| Vision Screening Required | New Drivers / Renewals |
| Renewal Format | In-Person / Mail-In |
| **Static Visual Acuity Requirements** | |
| Each Eye Without Correction | N/A |
| Both Eyes Without Correction | 20/40 |
| Each Eye With Correction | N/A |
| Both Eyes With Correction | 20/40 |
| If One Blind Eye – The other W/O Correction | 20/40 |
| If One Blind Eye – The other With Correction | 20/40 |
| *Absolute Visual Acuity Minimum (in each eye)* | **20/100** |
| Conditions | Each case is assessed before a medical board – Doctor's certificate required |
| **Visual Field Requirements** | No[*] |

| | |
|---|---|
| **Color Vision Requirement** | No |
| **Allow Restricted License** | Yes |
| Restrictions | Daytime; Weather; Radius limitation; No Interstate driving; Limitations to specific routes |
| **Allow Retesting** | Yes |
| Conditions | Depends on results; certain restrictions may apply |
| **Allow Bioptic Telescopes** | No |

[*]Class E & D only. CDL is excluded due to stricter federal rules.

146

# Maine

| License Renewal Procedures | |
|---|---|
| Renewal Intervals | 6 Years<br>4 Years (65+) |
| Vision Screening Required | New Drivers /<br>At age 40, 52, 65, and every Renewal after 62 |
| Renewal Format | Mail-In / In-Person |

| Visual Acuity Requirements | |
|---|---|
| Best Eye With / Without Correction | 20/40 |
| *Absolute Visual Acuity Minimum* | **20/70 in each eye** |

| Visual Field Requirement | |
|---|---|
| Both Eyes | 140° unrestricted |
| Both Eyes | 110° restricted |
| Visual Field Testing Method | Titmus II or Stereo Optical Vision Screening Equipment |

| Color Vision Requirement | No |
|---|---|
| **Allow Restricted License** | Yes |
| Conditions | Daytime only; Radius from Home; Special equipment (e.g., mirrors) |
| **Allow Retesting** | Yes |
| Conditions | Must be tested by an Eye Care Specialist |
| **Allow Bioptic Telescopes** | No |
| Offer Low Vision Driver's Training / Education | No |

# Maryland

| License Renewal Procedures | |
|---|---|
| Renewal Intervals | 5 Years |
| Vision Screening Required | New Drivers / Renewals |
| Renewal Format | In-Person |
| **Visual Acuity Requirements** | |
| Each Eye Without Correction | 20/40 |
| Both Eyes Without Correction | 20/40 |
| Each Eye With Correction | 20/40 |
| Both Eyes With Correction | 20/40 |
| If One Blind Eye – The other W/O Correction | 20/40 |
| If One Blind Eye – The other With Correction | 20/40 |
| *Absolute Visual Acuity Minimum* | **20/100** |
| **Comment** | Persons with Best corrected vision of 20/70 – 20/100 must be processed by HQ only |
| **Visual Field Requirement** | |
| Each Eye / Both Eyes | 70° (± 35°) / 110° (140° no restrictions) |
| Visual Field Testing Method | Stereo Optical Optec 1000 vision screener |

| Color Vision Requirement | Yes (commercial license only) |
|---|---|
| **Allow Restricted License** | Yes |
| Conditions | Daytime only; Outside mirrors for low vision drivers |
| **Allow Retesting if driver fails vision screening** | Yes |
| Conditions | Test by Eye Care Specialist; Checkup and Driving test by Occupational Therapist; Specialized driver training |
| **Allow Bioptic Telescopes** | Yes |
| Restrictions | Daytime only, Outside mirrors, Others possible |
| Absolute Corrected Minimum Through Telescope(s) | 20/70 |
| Absolute Corrected Minimum Through Carrier Lens | 20/100 |
| Require Special Bioptic Telescope Training / Test | Yes |
| Offer Low Vision Driver's Training / Education | Yes |

# Massachusetts

| License Renewal Procedures | |
|---|---|
| Renewal Interval | 5 Years |
| Vision Screening Required | New Drivers / Renewals |
| Renewal Format | In-Person |
| Mandatory Vision Test | Each Renewal |
| **Visual Acuity Requirements** | |
| Each Eye Without Correction | N/A |
| Both Eyes Without Correction | N/A |
| Each Eye With Correction | N/A |
| Either Eye With Correction | 20/40 |
| If One Blind Eye – The other W/O Correction | N/A |
| If One Blind Eye – The other With Correction | 20/40 |
| *Absolute Visual Acuity Minimum* | **20/70** (Daytime only) **20/100** (With bioptic) |
| **Visual Field Requirement** | |
| Each Eye / Both Eyes | 120° |
| Testing Method | Optec 1000 Vision Testing Machine |

| Color Vision Requirement | Yes (Distinguish Red, Green, Amber) |
|---|---|
| Allow Retesting if driver fails visual screening | Yes |
| **Allow Restricted License** | Yes |
| Conditions | Daytime |
| **Allow Bioptic Telescopes** | Yes |
| Restrictions | Daylight only, Mag. ≤ 3.0×, Fixed Focus |
| Absolute Corrected Minimum Through Telescope(s) | 20/40 |
| Absolute Corrected Minimum Through Carrier Lens | 20/100 in each eye |
| Require Special Bioptic Telescope Training / Test | No |
| Offer Low Vision Driver's Training / Education | No |

# Michigan

| License Renewal Procedures | |
|---|---|
| Renewal Interval | 4 Years |
| Vision Screening Required | New Drivers / Renewals |
| Renewal Format | Mail-in every other renewal |
| **Visual Acuity Requirements** | |
| Each Eye Without Correction | 20/40 |
| Both Eyes Without Correction | 20/40 |
| Each Eye With Correction | 20/40 |
| Both Eyes With Correction | 20/40 |
| If One Eye 20/100 or less The other W/O Correction | 20/50 |
| If One Eye 20/100 or less The other With Correction | 20/50 |
| *Absolute Visual Acuity Minimum* | **See next page** |
| **Visual Field Requirement** | |
| Both Eyes | 110°–140° – No restrictions 90° –110° – Restricted |
| Method of Testing | Tangent Screen, perimetry, 6 mm target |

| Color Vision | No |
|---|---|
| **Allow Restricted License** | Yes; **See next page** |
| **Allow Retesting if applicant fails first visual screening** | Yes |
| Conditions | None |
| **Allow Bioptic Telescopes** | Yes |
| Restrictions | Same as corrective Lens |
| Absolute Corrected Minimum Through Telescope(s) | Same as Vision Standard |
| Absolute Corrected Minimum Through Carrier Lens | No |
| Require Special Bioptic Telescope Training | Recommended |
| Require Special Bioptic Telescope Test | Recommended |

150

*Appendix E*

**Summary of Vision Screening Standards For Driver Licensing In Michigan**

Generally, drivers who meet screening requirements of 20/40 or better are granted full driving privileges unless a vision specialist recommends otherwise, or, other physical conditions require restrictions or denial of a license. Drivers who are screened at less than 20/40 fall into the following categories:

**Vision With No Progressive Abnormalities or Diseases of the Eye:**
1a. Less than 20/40 to and including 20/50 – full driving privileges
1b. Less than 20/50 to and including 20/70 – daylight driving only
1c. Less than 20/70 – not eligible for licensing

**Vision With Progressive Abnormalities or Diseases of the Eye:**
**(Cataracts, Glaucoma, AMD, RP, Other)**
1a. Less than 20/40 to and including 20/50 – full driving privileges
1b. Less than 20/50 to and including 20/60 – daylight driving only
1c. Less than 20/60 – not eligible for licensing

**Drivers With Vision 20/100 or Less in One Eye and the Other Eye as Follows:**
1a. Up to and including 20/50 – full driving privileges
1b. Less than 20/50 – not eligible for licensing

**Peripheral Vision:**
1a. 140° to and including 110° – full driving privileges
2b. Less than 110° to and including 90° – subject to additional conditions and requirements
3c. Less than 90° – not eligible for licensing

# Minnesota

| License Renewal Procedures | |
|---|---|
| Renewal Interval | 4 Years |
| Vision Screening Required | New Drivers / Renewals |
| Renewal Format | In-Person |
| **Visual Acuity Requirements** | |
| Each Eye Without Correction | N/A |
| Both Eyes Without Correction | N/A |
| Each Eye With Correction | N/A |
| Both Eyes With Correction | 20/40 |
| If One Blind Eye – The other W/O Correction | N/A |
| If One Blind Eye – The other With Correction | N/A |
| *Absolute Visual Acuity Minimum* | **20/80** |
| **Visual Field Requirement** | |
| Both Eyes | 105° |
| Visual Field Screening | New / Renewal / Professional |

| | |
|---|---|
| **Color Vision Requirement** | No |
| **Allow Restricted License** | Yes |
| Conditions | Daytime |
| **Allow Retesting if driver fails visual screening** | Yes |
| Conditions | None |
| **Allow Bioptic Telescopes** | No |
| **Provide Low Vision Drivers Training** | No |

152

# Mississippi

| License Renewal Procedures | |
|---|---|
| Renewal Interval | 4 Years |
| Vision Screening Required | New Drivers |
| Renewal Format | In-Person |
| **Visual Acuity Requirements** | |
| Each Eye Without Correction | 20/40 |
| Both Eyes With Correction | 20/40 |
| If One Blind Eye – The other With Correction | N/A |
| *Absolute Visual Acuity Minimum* | **20/70 daytime 20/200 TX** |
| **Visual Field Requirement** | |
| Both eyes | 140° No restrictions |
| One eye | T 70°; N 35° with 2 outside mirrors |

| Color Vision Requirement | No |
|---|---|
| **Allow Restricted License** | Yes |
| Conditions | Daytime |
| **Allow Retesting if Driver Fails First Screening** | Yes |
| Conditions | None |
| **Allow Bioptic Telescopes** | Yes |
| Absolute corrected Minimum through Telescope | 20/50 |
| Absolute corrected Minimum through Carrier Lens | 20/200 |
| Conditions | Central field loss ≤ 5°; Horizontal field ≥ 105° without expanders; telescope mag ≤ 4.0× |
| Offer Low Vision Driver's Training / Education | No |
| Require Special Bioptic Telescope Training / Test | Yes / Yes |

# Missouri

| License Renewal Procedures | |
|---|---|
| Renewal Interval | 6 Years |
| Vision Screening Required | New Drivers / Renewal |
| Renewal Format | In-Person, by mail if out of state. |

| Visual Acuity Requirements | |
|---|---|
| Each Eye Without Correction | 20/40 |
| Both Eyes Without Correction | 20/40 |
| Each Eye With Correction | 20/40 |
| Both Eyes With Correction | 20/50 |
| If One Blind Eye – The other W/O Correction | 20/50 |
| If One Blind Eye – The other With Correction | 20/50 |
| *Absolute Visual Acuity Minimum* | **20/160** |

| Visual Field Requirement | |
|---|---|
| Both eyes / Each eye / One eye only | 70° / 55° / 85° (requires mirror on other side) |
| Test Method | Objective / Quantitative |

| Color Vision Requirement | No |
|---|---|
| **Allow Restricted License** | Yes |
| Restrictions | 20/41 to 20/59 – Daylight 20/60 to 20/74 – Daylight, 45mph speed limit 20/41 to 20/59 – Road test + additional restrictions Better eye 50°–80° – Daylight, 45mph speed limit |
| **Allow Bioptic Telescopes** | Not for meeting vision requirements, but for driving |
| Restrictions | According to results of vision screening |
| Absolute Corrected Minimum Through Carrier Lens | 20/160 |
| Require Special Bioptic Telescope Training / Test | No |
| Offer Low Vision Driver's Training / Education | No |

# Montana

| License Renewal Procedures | |
|---|---|
| Renewal Interval | 8 Years, 4 Years 75+ |
| Vision Screening Required | New Drivers / Renewals |
| Renewal Format | Mail-In / In-Person |
| **Visual Acuity Requirements** | |
| Each Eye Without Correction | 20/40 |
| Both Eyes Without Correction | 20/40 |
| Each Eye With Correction | 20/40 |
| Both Eyes With Correction | 20/40 |
| If One Blind Eye – The other W/O Correction | 20/40 |
| If One Blind Eye – The other With Correction | 20/40 |
| *Absolute Visual Acuity Minimum* | **20/100** |
| **Visual Field Requirement** | (Commercial only) |
| Both Eyes | 70° |

| Color Vision Requirement | Commercial only |
|---|---|
| Allow Retesting if fails vision screening | Yes |
| Conditions | None |
| **Allow Restricted License** | Yes |
| Restrictions | Daytime; Weather; Season restrictions Speed Limit – 45mph; Interstate Speed Limit – 55mph |
| **Allow Bioptic Telescopes** | Yes |
| Restrictions | No Bioptics allowed during road test |
| Absolute Corrected Minimum Through Carrier Lens | 20/100 |
| Require Special Bioptic Telescope Training / Test | No |
| Offer Low Vision Driver's Training / Education | No |

# Nebraska

| License Renewal Procedures | |
|---|---|
| Renewal Interval | 5 Years |
| Vision Screening required | New Drivers / Renewals |
| Renewal Format | In-Person |

| Visual Acuity Requirements | |
|---|---|
| Each Eye Without Correction | 20/40* |
| Both Eyes Without Correction | 20/40* |
| Each Eye With Correction | 20/40* |
| Both Eyes With Correction | 20/40* |
| If One Blind Eye – The other W/O Correction | 20/40* |
| If One Blind Eye – The other With Correction | 20/40* |
| *Absolute Visual Acuity Minimum* | **20/70** ** |
| Restrictions | Daylight, outside mirrors, speed restriction |

| Visual Field Requirement | |
|---|---|
| Each Eye / Both Eyes | 70° / 140° |
| Exceptions both eyes | 100°–119° – Outside Mirrors 120°–130° – with Restrictions |
| Method used to test visual field | Vision Machine |

| Color Vision Requirement | Commercial only |
|---|---|
| **Allow Restricted License** | Yes |
| Conditions | Daytime |
| **Allow Bioptic Telescopes** | Yes |
| Restrictions | Annual Retest; vision and road test |
| Absolute Corrected Minimum Through Telescope(s) | 20/70 |
| Absolute Corrected Minimum Through Carrier Lens | N/A |
| Require Special Bioptic Telescope Training / Test | Annual Road Test |
| Offer Low Vision Driver's Training / Education | No |

*Higher reading acceptable with restrictions (Daylight only, outside mirrors, or both)

**The other eye not blind

# Nevada

| License Renewal Procedures | |
|---|---|
| Renewal Interval | 4 Years |
| Vision Screening required | New Drivers, In-Person Renewals |
| Renewal Format | In-Person (By mail every other renewal) |
| Mandatory Vision Test | After Age 70 |
| **Visual Acuity Requirements** | |
| Each Eye Without Correction | 20/40 |
| Both Eyes Without Correction | 20/40 |
| Each Eye With Correction | 20/40 |
| Both Eyes With Correction | 20/40 |
| If One Blind Eye – The other W/O Correction | 20/40 |
| If One Blind Eye – The other With Correction | 20/40 |
| *Absolute Visual Acuity Minimum* | **20/50**, other eye no worse than 20/60 – daylight driving only |
| **Visual Field Requirement** | |
| Each Eye / Both Eyes | 75° / 75° |

| | |
|---|---|
| **Color Vision Requirement** | No |
| **Allow Restricted License** | Yes |
| Conditions | Daytime only |
| **Allow retesting if fail vision screening** | Yes |
| **Allow Bioptic Telescopes** | Yes |
| Restrictions | Side mirrors; Annual retest; Daylight only; Speed limit; Annual vision and driving tests |
| Absolute Corrected Minimum Through Telescope(s) | 20/40 |
| Absolute Corrected Minimum Through Carrier Lens | 20/120 |
| Require Special Bioptic Telescope Training / Test | Yes, road test |
| Offer Low Vision Driver's Training / Education | No |

# New Hampshire

| License Renewal Procedures | |
|---|---|
| Renewal Interval | 4 Years |
| Vision Screening Required | New Drivers / Renewal / Duplicates |
| Renewal Format | In-Person / Mail-In |
| Driving Test Required at Age | 75 |
| **Visual Acuity Requirements** | |
| Each Eye Without Correction | 20/40 |
| Both Eyes Without Correction | 20/40 |
| Each Eye With Correction | 20/40 |
| Both Eyes With Correction | 20/40 |
| If One Blind Eye – The other W/O Correction | 20/30 |
| If One Blind Eye – The other With Correction | 20/30 |
| *Absolute Visual Acuity Minimum* | **20/70***|
| **Visual Field Requirement** | No |

| | |
|---|---|
| **Color Vision Requirement** | No |
| **Allow Retesting if fail screening** | Yes |
| Conditions | None |
| **Allow Restricted License** | Yes |
| Conditions | Daytime only |
| **Allow Bioptic Telescopes** | Yes |
| Restrictions | Daytime only |
| Absolute Corrected Minimum Through Telescope(s) | 20/30 |
| Absolute Corrected Minimum Through Carrier Lens | No |
| Require Special Bioptic Telescope Test | Yes |
| Offer Low Vision Driver's Training / Education | No |

*Between 20/50 to 20/70 could be restricted to operating during daylight hours only. The vision form must be completed by a medical doctor.

# New Jersey

| License Renewal Procedures | |
|---|---|
| Renewal Interval | 4 Years |
| Vision Screening Required | New Drivers |
| Renewal Format | Mail-In after age 21 |
| **Visual Acuity Requirements** | |
| Each Eye Without Correction | 20/50 |
| Both Eyes Without Correction | 20/50 |
| Each Eye With Correction | 20/50 |
| Both Eyes With Correction | 20/50 |
| If One Blind Eye – The other W/O Correction | 20/50 |
| If One Blind Eye – The other With Correction | 20/50 |
| *Absolute Visual Acuity Minimum* | **20/50** |
| **Visual Field Requirement** | No |

| Color Vision Requirement | Yes, new drivers (not cause for denial) |
|---|---|
| **Allow Retesting if fails visual screening** | Yes |
| Conditions | Applicant must attain minimum standard of 20/50 in one eye with device |
| **Allow Restricted License** | Yes |
| Conditions | Daytime only |
| **Allow Bioptic Telescopes** | Yes |
| Restrictions | Daylight only |
| Absolute Corrected Minimum Through Telescope(s) | 20/50 |
| Absolute Corrected Minimum Through Carrier Lens | Determine by director |
| Require Special Bioptic Telescope Test | Yes |
| Offer Low Vision Driver's Training / Education | No |

# New Mexico

| License Renewal Procedures | |
| --- | --- |
| Renewal Intervals | 4 or 8 Years<br>1 Year after age 75 |
| Vision Screening Required | New Drivers / Renewals |
| Renewal Format | In-Person |
| **Visual Acuity Requirements** | |
| Each Eye Without Correction | 20/40 |
| Both Eyes Without Correction | 20/40 |
| Each Eye With Correction | 20/40 |
| Both Eyes With Correction | 20/40 |
| If One Blind Eye – The other W/O Correction | 20/40 |
| If One Blind Eye – The other With Correction | 20/40 |
| *Absolute Visual Acuity Minimum* | 20/40 |
| **Visual Field Requirement** | Only if applicant fails vision screening |
| Testing Method | Normal Ophthalmic Procedures |

| Color Vision Requirement | No |
| --- | --- |
| **Allow Retesting if fails visual screening** | Yes |
| Conditions | Applicant must be tested by Eye Care Specialist |
| **Allow Restricted License** | Yes |
| Conditions | Daytime only; Radius from home; Annual renewal |
| **Allow Bioptic Telescopes** | No |
| Offer Low Vision Driver's Training / Education | No |

160

# New York

| License Renewal Procedures | |
|---|---|
| Renewal Interval | 5 Years |
| Vision Screening Required | New Drivers |
| Renewal Format | Mail-In / In-Person |
| **Visual Acuity Requirements** | |
| Each Eye Without Correction | N/A |
| Both Eyes Without Correction | 20/40 |
| Each Eye With Correction | N/A |
| Both Eyes With Correction | 20/40 |
| One Blind Eye – The other With or Without Correction | 20/40 |
| *Absolute Visual Acuity Minimum* | **Better than 20/70** one or both eyes; field of vision must be 140° |
| **Visual Field Requirement** | Only if vision less than 20/40 |

| Dynamic Acuity Test | N/A |
|---|---|
| **Color Vision Requirement** | No |
| **Allow Restricted License** | Yes |
| Restrictions | Daytime; Mirrors; Access to limited roads; Other restrictions are added based on eye care provider recommendations |
| **Allow Retesting** | Yes |
| **Allow Bioptic Telescopes** | Yes |
| Restrictions | Periodic Vision statement every 6 or 12 months |
| Absolute Corrected Minimum Through Telescope(s) | 20/40 |
| Absolute Corrected Minimum Through Carrier Lens | 20/100 |
| Require Bioptic Telescope Training / Driving Test | Yes / Yes |
| Offer Low Vision Driver's Training / Education | No |

## North Carolina

| License Renewal Procedures | |
|---|---|
| Renewal Interval | 5 Years |
| Vision Screening Required | New Drivers / Renewal |
| Renewal Format | In-Person |
| **Visual Acuity Requirements** | |
| Each Eye Without Correction | 20/40 |
| Both Eyes Without Correction | 20/40 |
| Each Eye With Correction | 20/50 |
| Both Eyes With Correction | 20/50 |
| If One Blind Eye – The other W/O Correction | 20/30 |
| If One Blind Eye – The other With Correction | 20/40 |
| *Absolute Visual Acuity Minimum* | **20/100** 20/70 if one eye blind |
| **Visual Field Requirement** | Commercial Only 70° in each eye |

| Color Vision Requirement | Commercial only |
|---|---|
| **Allow Retesting if fails visual screening** | Yes |
| Conditions | Eye Care Specialist test; Driving test |
| **Allow Restricted License** | Yes |
| Conditions | Daytime; Speed restrictions; No Interstate driving |
| **Allow Bioptic Telescopes** | No |
| Offer Low Vision Driver's Training / Education | No |

# North Dakota

| License Renewal Procedures | |
|---|---|
| Renewal Interval | 4 Years |
| Vision Screening Required | New Drivers / Renewals |
| Renewal Format | In-Person |
| Mandatory Vision Test | Each Renewal |
| **Visual Acuity Requirements** | |
| Both Eyes Without Correction | 20/40 |
| Both Eyes With Correction | 20/40 |
| If One Blind Eye – The other W/O Correction | 20/40 |
| If One Blind Eye – The other With Correction | 20/40 |
| *Absolute Visual Acuity Minimum* | **20/80 –** Better Eye **20/100 –** Worse Eye |
| **Visual Field Requirement** | |
| New / Professional / Renewal | |
| Each Eye / Both Eyes | 70° / 140° |
| Visual Field Test Method | OPTEC 1000 Vision Tester |

| Color Vision Requirement | Commercial only |
|---|---|
| **Allow Restricted License** | Yes |
| Conditions | Daytime; Pending a sight-related road test, Area and Distance Restriction may also be applied |
| **Allow Retesting** | Yes |
| **Allow Bioptic Telescopes** | Yes |
| Restrictions | Daytime only; Area; Speed Maximum; Annual Vision Report Required |
| Absolute Corrected Minimum Through Telescope(s) | 20/40 |
| Absolute Corrected Minimum Through Carrier Lens | 20/130 |
| Require Special Bioptic Telescope Training / Test | No |
| Offer Low Vision Driver's Training / Education | No |

# Ohio

| License Renewal Procedures | |
|---|---|
| Renewal Interval | 4 Years |
| Vision Screening Required | New Drivers / Renewals |
| Renewal Format | In-Person |
| **Visual Acuity Requirements** | |
| Each Eye Without Correction | 20/40 |
| Both Eyes Without Correction | 20/40 |
| Either Eye With Correction | 20/40 |
| Better Eye With or Without Correction | 20/40 |
| One Blind Eye – The other With/Without Correction | 20/30 |
| *Absolute Visual Acuity Minimum* | **20/70** |
| **Visual Field Requirement** | |
| New drivers / professionals / renewals | |
| Each eye / Both eyes | 70° / 140° (±70°) |
| Visual Field Testing Method | Keystone Vision II |

| | |
|---|---|
| **Color Vision Requirement** | Yes (for professional drivers) |
| **Allow Restricted License** | Yes |
| Conditions | Daytime |
| **Allow Retesting if Driver Fails First Screening** | Yes |
| Conditions | Retest by state-approved and contracted Eye Care Specialist |
| **Allow Bioptic Telescopes** | Yes |
| Restrictions | Daylight driving only for 1st year. Afterward, retest for day + night driving |
| Absolute Corrected Minimum Through Telescope(s) | 20/70 |
| Absolute Corrected Minimum Through Carrier Lens | 20/200 |
| Require Special Bioptic Telescope Training / Test | Yes / Yes |
| Offer Low Vision Driver's Training / Education | Yes* |

*See following page for Ohio addresses

For bioptic/telescopic vision evaluators contact:

**Greg Wood, O.D.**
**The Ohio State School of Optometry Low Vision Clinic**
**320 W 10th Ave, Columbus OH  43210**

For information on bioptic/telescopic driver training, contact:

**The Vision Center of Central Ohio**
**1393 N High St., Columbus OH  43201**

For information on bioptic/telescopic driver testing, contact:

**Driver License Manager Serge Baranowski**
**Office of Licensing and Commercial Standards Driver License Unit**
**1970 W Broad St., Columbus OH  43223**

# Oklahoma

| License Renewal Procedures | |
|---|---|
| Renewal Interval | 4 Years |
| Vision Screening Required | New Drivers |
| Renewal Format | Mail-In / In-Person |
| **Visual Acuity Requirements** | |
| Each Eye Without Correction | 20/60 |
| Both Eyes Without Correction | 20/60 |
| Each Eye With Correction | 20/60 |
| Both Eyes With Correction | 20/60 |
| If One Blind Eye – The other W/O Correction | 20/50 |
| If One Blind Eye – The other With Correction | 20/50 |
| *Absolute Visual Acuity Minimum* | **20/100** |
| **Visual Field Requirement** | |
| Each / Both Eyes | 30° / 30° |

| | |
|---|---|
| Allow Retesting after driver fails vision screening | Yes |
| **Allow Restricted License** | Yes |
| Conditions | Daytime; Speed limit; locale |
| **Allow Bioptic Telescopes** | No |

# Oregon

| License Renewal Procedures | |
|---|---|
| Renewal Interval | 8 Years |
| Vision Screening Required | New Drivers / Renewals – Age 50+ |
| Renewal Format | In-Person |
| **Visual Acuity Requirements** | |
| Each Eye Without Correction | 20/40 |
| Both Eyes Without Correction | 20/40 |
| Either Eye With Correction | 20/40 |
| Better Eye With or Without Correction | 20/40 |
| If One Blind Eye – The other With Correction | 20/40 |
| *Absolute Visual Acuity Minimum* | **20/70** |
| **Visual Field Requirement** | |
| Both Eyes | 110° |

| | |
|---|---|
| **Color Vision Requirement** | No |
| **Allow Restricted License** | Yes |
| Conditions | Daytime for vision between 20/40 and 20/70 |
| **Allow Retesting if Driver Fails First Screening** | Yes |
| **Allow Bioptic Telescopes** | Yes |
| Restrictions | Must pass vision test with carrier lens only |
| Absolute Corrected Minimum Through Telescope(s) | 20/40 |
| Absolute Corrected Minimum Through Carrier Lens | 20/40 20/70 – Daylight only |
| Require Special Bioptic Telescope Training / Test | No |
| Offer Low Vision Driver's Training / Education | No |

# Pennsylvania

| License Renewal Procedures | |
|---|---|
| Renewal Interval | 4 Years |
| Vision Screening Required | New Drivers |
| Renewal Format | In-Person |
| **Visual Acuity Requirements** | |
| Both Eyes Without Correction | 20/40 |
| One Blind Eye – The other Without Correction | 20/40 |
| If One Blind Eye – The other With Correction | 20/40 |
| *Absolute Visual Acuity Minimum* | **20/100** |
| **Visual Field Requirement** | New drivers, professionals |
| Both Eyes | 120° |

| | |
|---|---|
| **Color Vision Requirement** | No |
| **Allow Restricted License** | Yes |
| Conditions | Daytime; Area restriction; Mirrors; Class restriction |
| **Allow Retesting if Driver Fails First Screening** | N/A |
| **Allow Bioptic Telescopes** | Yes |
| Restrictions | Must pass vision test with carrier lens only. 20/100 at least |
| Require Special Bioptic Telescope Training / Test | Driving test and other restrictions |
| Offer Low Vision Driver's Training / Education | No |

# Rhode Island

| License Renewal Procedures | | Color Vision Requirement | No |
|---|---|---|---|
| Renewal Intervals | 5 Years; Age 68+ every 2 years | **Allow Restricted License** | No |
| | | **Allow Retesting** | Yes |
| Vision Screening Required | New Drivers / Renewals | **Allow Bioptic Telescopes** | No Idea[*] |
| Renewal Format | In-Person | Absolute Corrected Minimum Through Telescope(s) | N/A |
| **Visual Acuity Requirements** | | Absolute Corrected Minimum Through Carrier Lens | N/A |
| Each Eye Without Correction | 20/40 | Require Bioptic Telescope Training / Driving Test | N/A |
| Both Eyes Without Correction | 20/40 | Offer Low Vision Driver's Training / Education | No |
| Each Eye With Correction | 20/40 | | |
| Both Eyes With Correction | 20/40 | | |
| One Blind Eye – The other With or Without Correction | 20/40 | | |
| If One Blind Eye – The other With Correction | 20/40 | | |
| *Absolute Visual Acuity Minimum* | **20/40** | | |
| **Visual Field Requirement** | No | | |

[*]This was the response from the state's Department of Motor Vehicles to our questionnaire. Information from other sources indicates that as of 1995, bioptic telescopes are allowed in RI.

## South Carolina

| License Renewal Procedures | |
|---|---|
| Renewal Interval | 5 Years |
| Vision Screening Required | New Drivers / Renewals |
| Renewal Format | Mail-In / In-Person |
| **Visual Acuity Requirements** | |
| Each Eye Without Correction | 20/40 |
| Both Eyes Without Correction | 20/40 |
| Each Eye With Correction | 20/40 |
| Both Eyes With Correction | 20/40 |
| If One Blind Eye – The other With Correction | 20/40 |
| If One Blind Eye – The other W/O Correction | 20/40 – Must have outside mirror |
| *Absolute Visual Acuity Minimum* | **20/70** Better Eye, if other eye is better than 20/200 |
| **Visual Field Requirement** | No |

| Color Vision Requirement | No |
|---|---|
| **Allow Restricted License** | Yes |
| **Allow Retesting** | Yes |
| Conditions | None |
| **Allow Bioptic Telescopes** | Yes |
| Restrictions | No Bioptics allowed during vision test; Vision through carrier lens must meet state standards |
| Absolute Corrected Minimum Through Telescope(s) | N/A |
| Absolute Corrected Minimum Through Carrier Lens | 20/70 |
| Require Special Bioptic Telescope Training / Test | No |
| Offer Low Vision Driver's Training / Education | No |

# South Carolina

**If Worst Eye is Blind:**

20/200 or Worse – The better eye must be 20/40 or better to pass

**If the Worst Eye is Not Blind:**

20/200 or Better – The good eye must be 20/70 or better to pass

Out of State eye statements are acceptable only if all necessary information provided is comparable to information required on Form 412

Either eye scored worse than 20/40 without glasses, but both together score 20/70 or better with glasses, if needed – **Pass** – Restrict to glasses if needed

Both eyes together with BEST correction scores worse than 20/70 – **Fail**

One eye blind, other eye without glasses scores worse than 20/40 but with glasses 20/40 or better – **Pass** – Restrict to glasses

One eye blind, other eye with best correction scores worse than 20/40 – **Fail**

**Restrictions: Corrective Lens, Outside Mirrors, Daylight Driving Only**

# South Dakota

| License Renewal Procedures | |
|---|---|
| Renewal Interval | 5 Years |
| Vision Screening Required | New Drivers / Renewals |
| Renewal Format | In-Person |
| **Visual Acuity Requirements** | |
| Each Eye Without Correction | 20/50 |
| Both Eyes Without Correction | 20/40 |
| Each Eye With Correction | 20/50 |
| Both Eyes With Correction | 20/40 |
| If One Blind Eye – The other W/O Correction | 20/40 |
| If One Blind Eye – The other With Correction | 20/40 |
| *Absolute Visual Acuity Minimum* | **20/60** |
| **Visual Field Requirement** | No |

| | |
|---|---|
| Color Vision Requirement | No |
| **Allow Restricted License** | Yes |
| Restrictions | Daylight only; Outside rearview mirrors; Corrective lenses; 50 miles radius from home; No driving outside of town |
| **Allow Retesting** | Yes |
| Conditions | Obtain Eye Care Specialist vision statement |
| **Allow Bioptic Telescopes** | Yes |
| Restrictions | No rules. May use with a Bioptic lenses restriction |
| Absolute Corrected Minimum Through Telescope(s) | 20/40 |
| Absolute Corrected Minimum Through Carrier Lens | 20/40 20/60 – Restricted |
| Require Special Bioptic Telescope Training / Test | No |
| Offer Low Vision Driver's Training / Education | No |

# Tennessee

| License Renewal Procedures | |
|---|---|
| Renewal Interval | 5 Years |
| Vision Screening Required | New Drivers |
| Renewal Format | In-Person / Mail-In every other renewal |

| Visual Acuity Requirements | |
|---|---|
| Each Eye Without Correction | 20/40 |
| Both Eyes Without Correction | 20/40 |
| Each Eye With Correction | 20/40 |
| Both Eyes With Correction | 20/40 |
| If One Blind Eye – The other W/O Correction | 20/40 |
| If One Blind Eye – The other With Correction | 20/40 |
| *Absolute Visual Acuity Minimum* | **20/60** |

| Visual Field Requirement | (Professional drivers only) |
|---|---|
| Each eye / Both eyes | 70° / 70° |

| Color Vision Requirement | Yes (Professional drivers only) |
|---|---|
| **Allow Restricted License** | Yes |
| Restrictions | N/A |
| **Allow Retesting if driver fails visual screening** | No |
| **Allow Bioptic Telescopes** | Yes |
| Restrictions | Area limitation; annual medical update |
| Absolute Corrected Minimum Through Telescope(s) | 20/60 |
| Absolute Corrected Minimum Through Carrier Lens | 20/200 |
| Conditions | Visual field 150° or larger without expanders; Telescope power ≤ 4.0× |
| Require Special Bioptic Telescope Training / Test | Road Test during training |
| Offer Low Vision Driver's Training / Education | No (Low Vision Specialist provides training) |

# Texas

| License Renewal Procedures | |
|---|---|
| Renewal Interval | 6 Years |
| Vision Screening Required | New Drivers / Renewals (4, 5, 6 years) |
| Renewal Format – Eligible for alternate renewal if criteria is met | Alternate renewal by phone, mail or web |
| Visual Acuity Requirements | |
| Each Eye Without Correction | 20/40 |
| Both Eyes Without Correction | 20/40 |
| Best Eye With Correction | 20/50 |
| Both Eyes With Correction | 20/50 |
| If One Blind Eye – The other W/O Correction | 20/25 with eye specialist statement |
| If One Blind Eye – The other With Correction | 20/50 with eye specialist statement |
| Visual Acuity Minimum (if worse, case by case) | 20/70 – Daytime only; 45mph speed limit (no freeway) |
| Visual Field Requirement | No |

| Color Vision Requirement | Yes (all new drivers) & all commercial renewals |
|---|---|
| Allow Restricted License | Yes |
| Restrictions | Daytime only; Speed limit <45mph; No expressway driving; Any other advisable |
| Allow Retesting if driver fails visual screening | Yes |
| Conditions | Obtain a certificate from Eye Specialist; case by case basis |
| Allow Bioptic Telescopes | Yes |
| Restrictions | Case by case basis |
| Absolute Corrected Minimum Through Telescope(s) | 20/40 |
| Absolute Corrected Minimum Through Carrier Lens | Subject to review by medical board |
| Require Special Bioptic Telescope Test | Road Test |
| Offer Low Vision Driver's Training / Education | No |

# Utah

| License Renewal Procedures | |
|---|---|
| Renewal Interval | 5 Years |
| Vision Screening Required | New Drivers / Renewals: Age 65+ |
| Renewal Format | Mail-In every other renewal |
| **Visual Acuity Requirements** | |
| Each Eye Without Correction | 20/40 |
| Both Eyes Without Correction | 20/40 |
| Each Eye With Correction | 20/40 |
| Both Eye With Correction | 20/40 |
| If One Blind Eye – The other W/O Correction | 20/40 |
| If One Blind Eye – The other With Correction | 20/40 |
| *Absolute Visual Acuity Minimum* | **20/100** – in better eye |
| **Visual Field Requirement** | |
| Each eye / Both eyes On renewals | 120° / 120° (90° with restrictions) |
| Visual Field Testing Method | Stereo Optical (DMV2000) |

| Color Vision Requirement | Commercial drivers only |
|---|---|
| **Allow Restricted License** | Yes |
| Restrictions | Daytime only; Speed limit <45mph; radius limit |
| **Allow Retesting if driver fails visual screening** | Yes |
| Conditions | Three attempts allowed; Obtain a certificate from Eye Specialist |
| **Allow Bioptic Telescopes** | No |

## Vermont

| License Renewal Procedures | |
|---|---|
| Renewal Interval | 2 or 4 Years |
| Vision Screening Required | New Drivers |
| Renewal Format | Mail-In |
| **Visual Acuity Requirements** | |
| Each Eye Without Correction | N/A |
| Both Eyes Without Correction | 20/40 |
| Each Eye With Correction | N/A |
| Both Eyes With Correction | 20/40 |
| If One Blind Eye – The other W/O Correction | 20/40 |
| If One Blind Eye – The other With Correction | 20/40 |
| *Absolute Visual Acuity Minimum* | **20/40** |
| **Visual Field Requirement** | **New drivers** |
| Each Eye / Both Eyes | 60° / 60° |

| Color Vision Requirement | No |
|---|---|
| **Allow Restricted License** | Yes: for glasses or contact lenses |
| Allow Retesting | Yes: Applicant can submit an eyesight evaluation |
| **Allow Bioptic Telescopes** | Yes |
| Restrictions | Daytime only Under 10,000 lbs. |
| Absolute Corrected Minimum Through Telescope(s) | 20/40 |
| Absolute Corrected Minimum Through Carrier Lens | 20/40 |
| Require Special Bioptic Telescope Training / Test | Road Test Required |
| Offer Low Vision Driver's Training / Education | No |

# Virginia

| License Renewal Procedures | |
|---|---|
| Renewal Interval | 5 Years |
| Vision Screening Required | New Drivers / Renewals |
| Renewal Format | In-Person |
| **Visual Acuity Requirements** | |
| Each Eye Without Correction | 20/40 |
| Both Eyes Without Correction | 20/40 |
| Each Eye With Correction | 20/40 |
| Both Eyes With Correction | 20/40 |
| If One Blind Eye – The other W/O Correction | 20/40 |
| If One Blind Eye – The other With Correction | 20/40 |
| *Absolute Visual Acuity Minimum* | 20/70 daylight only |
| **Visual Field Requirement** | |
| Each Eye / Both Eyes | 100° / 100°. 70° / 70° – daylight only. One blind eye 40°T /30°N |
| Visual Field Testing Method | Stereo Optical / Titmus 10mm W @ 333mm |

| Color Vision Requirement | No |
|---|---|
| **Allow Retesting if applicant fails vision screening** | Yes |
| Conditions | Applicant can submit an eyesight evaluation by an Eye Care Specialist |
| **Allow Restricted License** | Yes |
| Restrictions | Daytime driving only |
| **Allow Bioptic Telescopes** | Yes |
| Restrictions | Daytime only for 1 year; After 1 year may take night driving test. Field 70° or better. |
| Absolute Corrected Minimum Through Telescope(s) | 20/70 |
| Absolute Corrected Minimum Through Carrier Lens | 20/200 |
| Require Special Bioptic Telescope Training / Test | Test Required |
| Offer Low Vision Driver's Training / Education | No |

# Washington

| License Renewal Procedures | |
|---|---|
| Renewal Interval | 5 Years |
| Vision Screening Required | New Drivers / Renewals |
| Renewal Format | In-Person |
| **Visual Acuity Requirements** | |
| Each Eye Without Correction | N/A |
| Both Eyes Without Correction | 20/40 |
| Each Eye With Correction | N/A |
| Both Eyes With Correction | 20/40 |
| If One Blind Eye – The other W/O Correction | 20/40 |
| If One Blind Eye – The other With Correction | 20/40 |
| *Absolute Visual Acuity Minimum* | **20/60** |
| **Visual Field Requirement** | |
| Each Eye / Both Eyes | 110° / 110° |
| Visual Field Testing Method | OPTEC 1000; Keystone Telebinocular; Keystone DVS II |

| Color Vision Requirement | Yes (for New and Professional drivers) |
|---|---|
| **Allow Retesting if applicant fails vision screening** | Yes |
| Conditions | Depends on situation |
| **Allow Restricted License** | Yes |
| Restrictions | Daytime driving only; Corrective lenses; Area limit; Outside mirrors |
| **Allow Bioptic Telescopes** | Yes |
| Restrictions | Depends on situation |
| Absolute Corrected Minimum Through Telescope(s) | N/A |
| Absolute Corrected Minimum Through Carrier Lens | N/A |
| Require Special Bioptic Telescope Training / Test | Training and Test Required |
| Offer Low Vision Driver's Training / Education | No |

*Appendix E*

# West Virginia

| License Renewal Procedures | |
|---|---|
| Renewal Interval | 5 Years |
| Vision Screening Required | New Drivers |
| Renewal Format | In-Person |
| **Visual Acuity Requirements** | |
| Each Eye Without Correction | N/A |
| Both Eyes Without Correction | 20/40 |
| Each Eye With Correction | N/A |
| Both Eyes With Correction | 20/40 |
| If One Blind Eye – The other W/O Correction | 20/40 |
| If One Blind Eye – The other With Correction | 20/40 |
| *Absolute Visual Acuity Minimum* | **20/60**[*] |
| **Visual Field Requirement** | No |

| | |
|---|---|
| **Color Vision Requirement** | No |
| **Allow Retesting if applicant fails vision screening** | Yes |
| Conditions | Applicant should submit an eyesight evaluation by an Eye Care Specialist |
| **Allow Restricted License** | No |
| **Allow Bioptic Telescopes** | No |
| Offer Low Vision Driver's Training / Education | No |

[*]If visual acuity below 20/20 the DMV Medical Advisory Board may consider peripheral vision, depth perception, and color recognition.

# Wisconsin

| License Renewal Procedures | |
|---|---|
| Renewal Interval | 8 Years |
| Vision Screening Required | New Drivers / Renewals |
| Renewal Format | In-Person |
| Mandatory Vision Test | Each Renewal |
| In-Person Renewal after Age | 70+ |

| Visual Acuity Requirements | |
|---|---|
| 20/40 In **Best** eye – with or without correction | |
| *Absolute Visual Acuity Minimum* | **20/100** |

| Visual Field Requirement | New / Professional / Renewal |
|---|---|
| Visual Field Test Method | Stereo optical machines |
| Each Eye / Both Eyes | 70° in **Best** Eye |

| Color Vision Requirement | Yes (professional drivers only) |
|---|---|
| **Allow Restricted License** | Yes |
| Conditions | Daytime; Mileage Restriction; Speed and/or Freeway Restriction; Mirrors |
| **Allow Retesting** | Yes |
| Condition | Referred to Vision Specialist |
| **Allow Bioptic Telescopes** | No |
| Offer Low Vision Driver's Training / Education | No |

# Wyoming

| License Renewal Procedures | |
|---|---|
| Renewal Interval | 4 Years |
| Vision Screening Required | New Drivers / Renewals |
| Renewal Format | Mail-In every other renewal |

| Visual Acuity Requirements | |
|---|---|
| Each Eye Without Correction | 20/40 |
| Both Eyes Without Correction | 20/40 |
| Each Eye With Correction | 20/40 |
| Both Eyes With Correction | 20/40 |
| If One Blind Eye – The other W/O Correction | 20/40 |
| If One Blind Eye – The other With Correction | 20/40 |
| *Absolute Visual Acuity Minimum* | **20/100** |

| Visual Field Requirement | |
|---|---|
| Both Eyes | 120° |
| Visual Field Screening | New, Renewal, Pro |
| Method of Testing | Keystone machine |

| Color Vision Requirement | No |
|---|---|
| **Allow Restricted License** | Yes |
| Conditions | Daytime; Weather; Season; Distance (usually) |
| **Allow Retesting** | Yes |
| Condition | Must show improvement before allowed another driving test |
| **Allow Bioptic Telescopes** | Yes |
| Restrictions | Distance restriction for at least one year |
| Absolute Corrected Minimum Through Telescope(s) | No – considered case by case |
| Absolute Corrected Minimum Through Carrier Lens | 20/100 both lenses |
| Require Special Bioptic Telescope Training / Test | Test only |
| Offer Low Vision Driver's Training / Education | No |

# APPENDIX F
# BIBLIOGRAPHY

Appel, S. D., Brilliant, R. L. and Reich, L. N. (1990). Driving with visual impairment: Facts and issues. *Journal of Vision Rehabilitation* **4**, 19–31.

Bailey (1987). Critical view of an ocular telephoto system. *Contact Lens Association of Ophthalmologists Journal* **13**, 217–221.

Ball, K., Owsley, C. and Beard, B. (1990). Clinical visual perimetry underestimates peripheral field problems in older adults. *Clin. Vision Sci.* **5**, 113–125.

Ball, K., Owsley, C., Sloane, M. E., Roenker, D. L. and Bruni, J. (1993). Visual attention problems as predictors of vehicle crashes in older drivers. *Invest. Ophthalmol. Vis. Sci.* **34(11)**, 3110–3122.

Burg, A. (1967). The relationship between vision test scores and driving record: General findings (Report 68–27): University of California, Los Angeles, Department of Engineering.

Chang, C. C. and Werner, K. (1999). Varitronix: An engineer's fairy tale. Information Display **4&5**, 38–40.

Charman, W. N. (1997). Vision and driving — A literature review and commentary. *Ophthal. Physiol. Opt.* **17**, 371–391.

Choyce, P. (1964). Galilean telescope using the anterior chamber implant as an eye-piece: a low visual-acuity aid for macular lesions. *Intra-Ocular Lenses and Implants*, H.K. Lewis & Co., London, 156–161.

Decina, L. E. and Staplin, L. (1993). Retrospective evaluation of alternative vision screening criteria for older and younger drivers. *Accident Analysis & Prevention* **25**, 267–275.

Demers-Turco, P. (1996). Driving with vision loss: Current issues in the United States. *Practical Optometry* **7(4)**, 143–148.

Donn, A. and Koester, C. J. (1986). An ocular telephoto system designed to improve vision in macular disease. *CLAO Journal* **12**, 81–85.

Filderman, I. P. (1959). The telecon lens for the partially-sighted. *Am. J. Optom. and Arch. Am. Acad. of Optom.* **36**, 135–136.

Foley, D. J., Wallace, R. B. and Eberhard, J. (1995). Risk factors for motor vehicle crashes among older drivers in a rural community. *Journal of the American Geriatric Society* **43**, 776–781.

Hilton, L. (2001). Study sparks laser eye surgery debate. *Review of Refractive Surgery* **January**, 10–13.

Huss, C. (1996). *West Virginia Low Vision Driving Study 1985-1995, Results and Conclusions*: West Virginia Division of Rehabilitation Services, West Virginia Rehabilitation Center.

Johnson, C. A. and Keltner, J. L. (1983). Incidence of visual field loss in 20,000 eyes and its relationship to driving performance. *Archives of Ophthalmology* **101**, 371–375.

Jose, R. T., Carter, K. and Carter, C. (1983). A training program for clients considering the use of bioptic telescope for driving. *J. of Visual Impairment and Blindness* **77**, 425–428.

Karmel, M. (2000). In the driver's seat. *Eye Net* **4**, 36–41.

Keltner, J. L. and Johnson, C. A. (1987). Visual function, driving safety, and the elderly. *Ophthalmology* **94**, 1180–1188.

Koziol, J. E., Peyman, G. A., Cionni, R., Chou, J.-S., Portney, V., Sun, R. and Tretacost, D. (1994). Evaluation and implementation of a teledioptric lens system for cataract and age-related macular degeneration. *Ophthalmic Surgery* **25**, 675–684.

Lipshitz, I., Loewenstein, A., Reingewirtz, M. and Lazar, M. (1997). An intraocular telescopic lens for macular degeneration. *Ophthalmic Surgery and Lasers* **28**, 513–517.

Lovsund, P., Hedin, A. and Tornros, J. (1991). Effects on driving performance of visual field defects: a driving simulator study. *Accid Anal Prev* **23**, 331–342.

Mackie, S. W., Webb, L. A., Hutchison, B. M., Hammer, H. M., Barrie, T. and Walsh, G. (1995). How much blame can be placed on laser photocoagulation for failure to attain driving standards? *Eye* **9**, 517–525.

McCloskey, L. W., Koepsell, T. D., Wolf, M. E. and Buchner, D. M. (1994). Motor vehicle collision injuries and sensory impairments of older drivers. *Age and Ageing* **23**, 267–273.

Moore, L. (1964). The contact lens for subnormal visual acuity. *British Journal of Physiological Optics* **21**, 203–204.

North, R. V. (1985). The relationship between the extent of visual field and driving performance — a review. *Ophthalmic Physiol Opt* **5**, 205–210.

Owsley, C. and Ball, K. (1993). Assessing visual function in the older driver. *Clinics in Geriatric Medicine* **9(2)**, 389–401.

Owsley, C., Ball, K., McGwin, G., Sloane, M. E., Roenker, D. L., White, M. F. and Overley, E. T. (1998). Visual processing impairment and risk of motor vehicle crash among older adults. *Jama* **279**, 1083–1088.

Owsley, C., Ball, K., Sloane, M. E., Roenker, D. L. and Bruni, J. R. (1991). Visual/Cognitive correlates of vehicle accidents in older drivers. *Psychology and Aging* **6**, 403–415.

Owsley, C. and McGwin, G., Jr. (1999). Vision impairment and driving. *Survey of Ophthalmology* **43**, 535–550.

Owsley, C., Stalvey, B., Wells, J. and Sloane, M. E. (1999). Older drivers and cataract: driving habits and crash risk. *Journals of Gerontology Series A, Biological Sciences and Medical Sciences* **54**, M203–M211.

Parisi, J. L., Bell, R. A. and Yassein, H. (1991). Homonymous hemianopic field defects and driving in Canada. *Can J Ophthalmol* **26**, 252–256.

Park, W. L., Unatin, J. and Hebert, A. (1993). A driving program for the visually impaired. *J. Am. Optom Assoc.* **64(1)**, 54–59.

Pearson, A. R., Tanner, V., Keightley, S. J. and Casswell, A. G. (1998). What effect does laser photocoagulation have on driving visual fields in diabetics? *Eye* **12**, 64–68.

Peli, E. (2000). Field expansion for homonymous hemianopia by optically-induced peripheral exotropia. *Optometry and Visual Science* **77**, 453–464.

Peli, E., Lipshitz, I. and Dotan, G. (2000). Implantable miniaturized telescope (IMT) for low vision. In C. Stuen, A. Arditi, A. Horowitz, M. A. Lang, B. Rosenthal and K. Seidman (Eds.), *Vision Rehabilitation: Assessment, Intervention and Outcomes*, Swets & Zeitlinger, Lisse, 200–203.

Szlyk, J. P., Seiple, W., Laderman, D. J., Kelsch, R., Ho, K. and McMahon, T. (1998). Use of bioptic amorphic lenses to expand the visual field in patients with peripheral loss. *Optometry and Vision Science* **75**, 518–524.

Transportation, U. S. D. of (1996). *National Highway Traffic Safety Administration: Traffic Safety Facts.*

Vingrys, A. J. and Cole, B. L. (1988). Are color vision standards justified in the transport industry? *Ophthal. Physiol. Opt.* **8**, 257–274.

Vogel, G. L. (1991). Training the bioptic telescope wearer for driving. *Bioptic telescopic spectacles for motor vehicle driving JAOA* **62**, 288–293.

Willis, T. R. and Portney, V. (1989). Preliminary evaluation of the Koziol-Peyman teledioptric system for age-related macular degeneration. *European Journal of Implant Refractive Surgery* **1**, 271–276.

Wood, J. M. and Troutbeck, R. (1992). Effect of restriction of the binocular visual field on driving performance. *Ophthal. Physiol. Opt.* **12**, 291–298.

# INDEX